From SLIGHT
to MIGHT

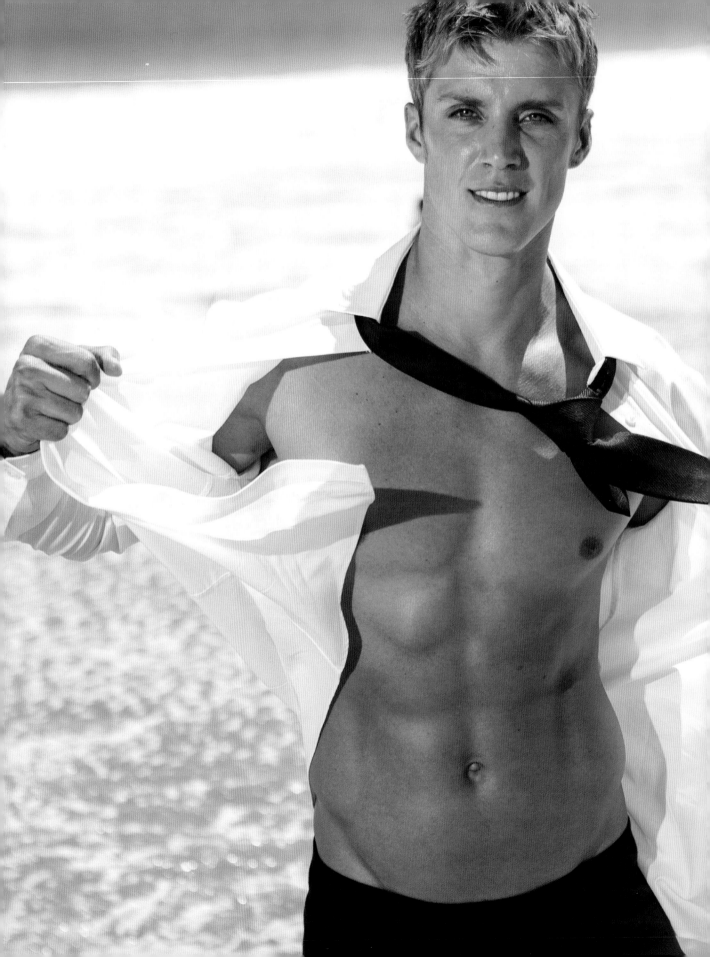

From SLIGHT to MIGHT

BUILDING MUSCLE FOR THE HARDGAINER

Hollis Lance Liebman

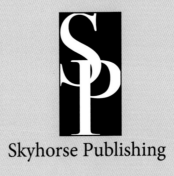

Skyhorse Publishing

General Disclaimer
The contents of this book are intended to provide useful information to the general public. All materials, including texts, graphics, and images, are for informational purposes only and are not a substitute for medical diagnosis, advice, or treatment for specific medical conditions. All readers should seek expert medical care and consult their own physicians before commencing any exercise program or for any general or specific health issues. The author and publishers do not recommend or endorse specific treatments, procedures, advice, or other information found in this book and specifically disclaim all responsibility for any and all liability, loss, or risk, personal or otherwise, which is incurred as a consequence, directly or indirectly, of the use or application of any of the material in this publication.

Visit our website at www.skyhorsepublishing.com.

10 9 8 7 6 5 4 3 2 1

Library of Congress Cataloging-in-Publication Data is available on file.

Cover design by Tom Lau
Project and art direction by Lisa Purcell Editorial & Design
Cover photographs by Jenn Schmidt Photography

Print ISBN: 978-1-5107-0895-2
Ebook ISBN: 978-1-5107-0897-6

Printed in China

CONTENTS

CONTENTS

SKINNY NO MORE

Y ou've probably seen those vintage Charles Atlas ads that show a muscle-bound bully kicking sand into the face of a scrawny guy who is just trying to enjoy a day at the beach with his girlfriend. The poor "skinny scarecrow" loses the girl, but he finds a book, one that will show him how to build muscles.

Do you see yourself in that skinny scarecrow? *Skinny, runt, pipsqueak, scrawny, weakling . . .* on and on go the labels you've heard all your life. You're on a lifelong pursuit for acceptance—and to simply fill out a shirt. Outsiders just never understand the burden you bear. As a kid you were ridiculed for your lack of size. You were likely the first to be picked on physically and the last to be picked for a team.

The tables turned as you got older, though. Your peers began to look at you with envy rather than ridicule. Although you are still slight in build and frame, it would seem nearly all of them have ballooned up and no longer

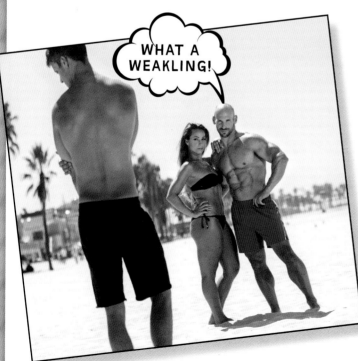

WHAT A WEAKLING!

bear much resemblance to the muscular and shapely youths they once were. Now they say, "You're so lucky! You can eat whatever you want and not gain weight."

"Yes," you reply, *"that's* the problem!"

To the world, you are known as the ectomorph, the hardgainer, but among others of your body type, you call yourself the tireless, the frustrated, the unfulfilled. And if you are one of the many ectomorphs who want to bulk up, you are, quite simply, the unfinished.

The other somatotypes (the mesomorphs and the endomorphs) may think that they envy you, but what they fail to realize is that you suffer an ongoing and most private of wars. A war of seclusion, avoidance, and embarrassment. And yes, while many ectos display somewhat prominent abdominals year-round, the cold, hard truth is you would give nearly anything to rip your shirt off to show off broad shoulders, a wide back, a thick chest, and arms that actually fill out shirts. Or at least a shoulder-width measurement that doesn't run parallel with your waistline.

Dare to dream.

Is there an ectomorph out there who hasn't thought about bulking up like the skinny guy does in those Charles Atlas ads? If only real life could imitate art, with you finally fulfilling your hidden muscular potential. You would thwart the bully and leave with the girl in the final frame. Alas, what is the steep price of admission to achieve that reality?

Just imagine for an instant that you, the ectomorph, the hardgainer, could truly defy your genetics and achieve your physique dreams. What if from now on, when someone looks your way, the thought "skinny" is replaced with "muscular"? What might that reality be worth to you?

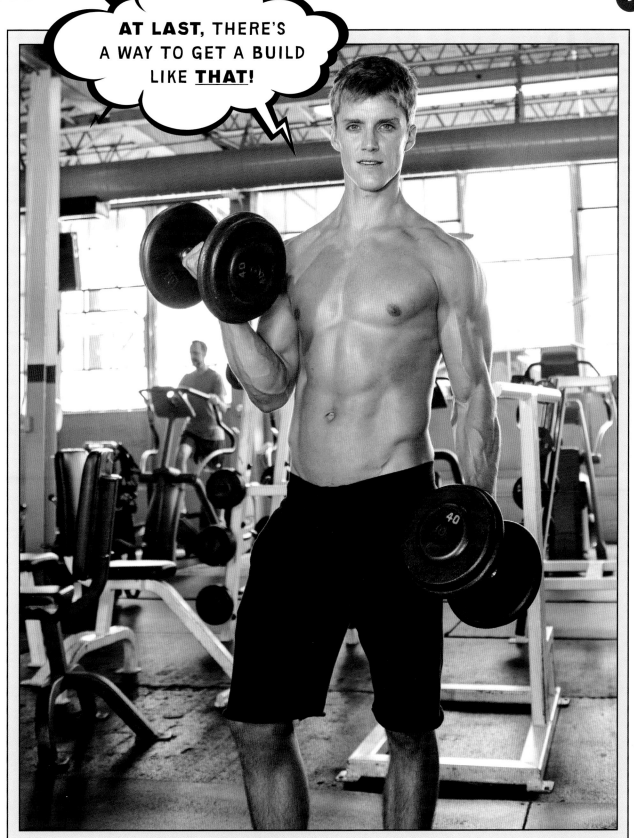

THE ECTO DILEMMA

In high school, I had a friend who was so completely over his ectomorph status and the thought of being relegated to skinny for life that he decided to do something about it. He piled on multiple layers of clothing to give the illusion to others—especially during gym class—that he was bigger than previously advertised. And with a newly revised diet of high protein and fat intake, progressive weight training and, of course, Father Time, within months the clothing layers (to give the illusion of muscles) were replaced with muscular layers.

Naturally this increase in size came with a price. He was constantly eating and would carry around his gallon of water all day while roaming the hallways going from class to class. Nevertheless, he had, to many sets of eyes—including mine—overcome his ectomorphic limitations. He wanted it bad enough that he defied genetics, taking matters into his own iron-forged hands, and won. Quite an achievement—especially for a young and impressionable kid. But the only impression left was on us, his classmates, who witnessed firsthand that transformation was possible, at any age and for any body type. At long last, an ecto had made it, had filled out his shirt. At long last, hardgainers had hope!

And then, just like that, all of his new gains disappeared. His pumped-up body seemed to deflate, leaving behind the original "skinny." Was it all just a dream or a terrible lie? Indeed, he *was* onto something. It was possible. It could be done. Now all he had to do was figure how to keep it done.

NO MORE FRUSTRATION

The pursuit of muscles isn't easy for a hardgainer. Frustration is a constant companion. So much so that many hardgainers decide to switch gears to pursue an endurance sport like marathon running or a triathlon. These are superb training modalities, but the participants are generally not known for their chiseled physiques with full and rippling musculature. Still others take a more drastic and permanent step: they simply give up, pulling themselves from the front lines of hope and change.

I am here to proclaim loudly that there is no need to give up, switch gears, or even curse genetics. The hardgainer's mission simply needs to be defined as "maximizing genetics." You cannot change the shape of your muscles, but you do have control over their composition, as well as their size. Will you ultimately have 20-inch arms and impressive thighs with more taper than a pyramid? It's possible . . . but most likely not. But will the reflection that stares back at you in the mirror instill a smile instead of a frown? Unequivocally, yes.

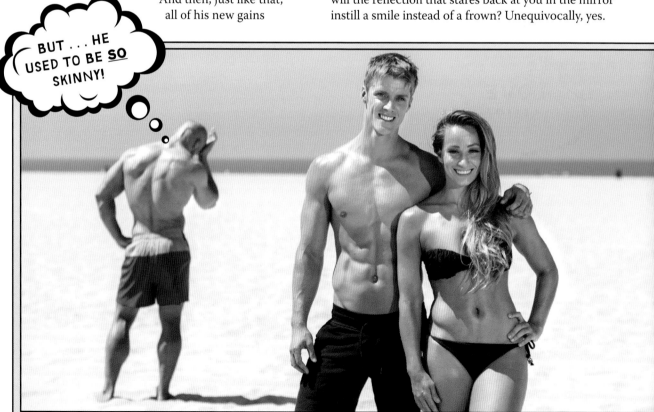

BUT . . . HE USED TO BE **SO** SKINNY!

Browse through any bookstore, discount warehouse, or online retailer and bear witness to dozens upon dozens of books on weight loss through every conceivable methodology known to humanity. Yet there is scant trace of books catering to the just as real and pertinent issues at hand for the hardgainer . . . until now.

The days of bulking up, marathon-like training, and excessive eating in the hopes of filling out are all but extinct. Providing an updated and revised resource on building the hardgainer for the twenty-first century, while retaining the trademark muscular quality and vascularity, is the goal of this book. What you hold in your hands is the manual and real-world plan written for you and your unique genetics and, ultimately, your breakthrough.

THE ECTOMORPH DEFINED

Just what is an ectomorph? As mentioned, there are three classifications of builds, or somatotypes, in which to categorize the human body: mesomorphic, endomorphic, and ectomorphic. Few of us fall neatly into just one of these categories—we tend to be a mixture of two—but generally one will be dominant.

Mesomorphs are predisposed to carrying lean muscle mass, and they possess naturally wide clavicles, a medium bone structure, and low body-fat levels. Many elite athletes fall within this classification.

Endomorphs are predisposed to storing body fat, and they possess a wide waist and shoulders, a large bone structure, and higher body-fat levels. People following a seemingly ongoing diet, who are prey to the yo-yo syndrome that comes with gaining and losing body fat for a lifetime, tend to be classified here.

And then there are the ectomorphs. Characterized by a narrow waist and clavicle structure, they tend to have speedy metabolisms and are thin not only from the front and back, but also from the side. Ectos generally carry long-limbed muscles, and they are not predisposed to packing on bulky muscle or body fat. Indeed, they can seemingly eat whatever they want, whenever they want, and not gain any appreciable weight. Yet their greatest blessing (a speedy metabolism) is also their greatest curse.

Ectomorphs seem to have a short list of undesirable qualities. Yet, although many are traditionally "skinny," not all can truly eat what they want and showcase a rippling midsection year round. Some ectos are what is commonly known as "skinny-fat," displaying not only a lightness in musculature but also an abundance of adipose (or fat), which makes for a rather petite and fleshy person. The jeans size may sound flattering, but it is the quality of the physique underneath the denim that tells a much bigger—and truer—story.

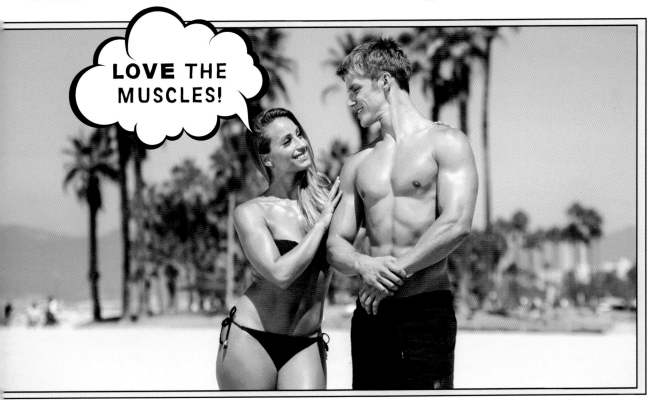

THE PLAN OVERVIEW

If you are an ectomorph, your journey to optimal fitness won't be easy—you must stay the course in the continuous belief that perseverance will overcome genetic limitations. Your blueprints are unique and differ from both endomorphs and mesomorphs, and, as such, they require a unique methodology.

On paper it would seem that your general approach would be a strict reliance on an almost overabundance of food and super heavy weights. But, like most things in life, there's more to it than that. Both the digestive system and the joints can handle only so much, so a surplus of nutrients and iron can actually be counterproductive to the acquisition of lean body mass. Excess calories beyond body maintenance and activity levels are generally stored as body fat, or in the case of the ectomorph, might simply be burned off through a superfast and ultra-efficient metabolism. Perhaps never more than here, the old adage "more is better" must be replaced with "better is better."

In addition, although you must lift progressively heavier weights to gradually gain solid muscle mass, relying solely on the sheer amount of weight you lift, coupled with your maximum lifting attempts (singles), does not yield larger musculature. A certain amount of momentum, joints, and muscles are working together to lift said poundage. In other words, the very low repetitions (one to three) employed by power lifters are effective for strength increases, but not for body-weight increases. What you have in common with the power lifter or strength-training athlete is that you all utilize multiple muscle groups to move an existing load. For example, during the bench press, although the pectorals are the key muscles firing, the triceps and anterior deltoids supply ancillary assistance. All these muscles working together is what allows you to move the maximum amount of weight (along with six to eight repetitions) and thus stimulate maximum muscle growth.

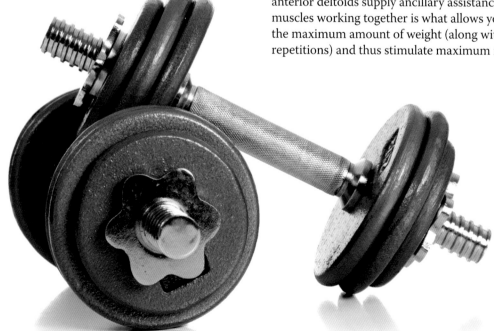

THE ECTO PRINCIPLES

What I have identified are six principles that, when consistently applied, will guide you on your journey to a stronger and fuller body, ultimately helping you to fulfill your dream of filling out a T-shirt in all the right places.

1. **Remain consistent.** In training, consistently sound nutrition and adequate recuperation will always deliver results. It is of little cumulative value to "be perfect" one day only to miss meals and training the next. You must remain consistent so that your vision at the beginning of the journey will become reality down the road. (Keep in mind that life happens, and you may miss a day. Even if you slip up, make sure to keep at it. After all, it's a marathon, not a sprint!)

2. **Reconfigure a raging metabolism.** The ectomorph's metabolic rate (the rate at which the body converts calories into energy) is usually fast—sometimes very fast. You must consistently overload on calories so that added weight sticks, but what is crucial is the quality of those calories. The ectomorph is doing himself a disservice by consuming an egg white omelet that, although high in muscle-building protein, is devoid of fat and at best contains trace elements. It will most likely leave him hungry again soon thereafter and "flattish" appearing in his muscles. Fats in the form of avocados, olive oils, salmon, and steak are the type that satiate hunger and bind and build muscle. More on this later.

3. **Learn the basics.** In building the ectomorph, multi-joint exercises, such as deadlifts and rows, should form the cornerstone of movements, which are akin to the foundation, whereas lateral raises and leg extensions are the decorations that enhance the previously laid structure. Form the structure first and furnish it later.

4. **Progressive resistance.** To stimulate muscle growth, you must progressively challenge your body. An arm that consistently curls 40 pounds for 6 to 8 repetitions will look the same. But upgrade to curling 50 pounds for the same number of repetitions, and it has been subjected to a new stimulus and will have no choice (through proper nutrition and rest) but to adapt by growing.

5. **Perform the right number of reps.** Along with progressive resistance, determining the correct number of repetitions per a given set is just as important as how they are performed. Too few (1 to 3) overly stresses the joints, too many (15 to 20) results in more of a cardio effect. For muscle growth, the lower body responds best to 8 to 12 repetitions and the upper body 6 to 10. More on this later.

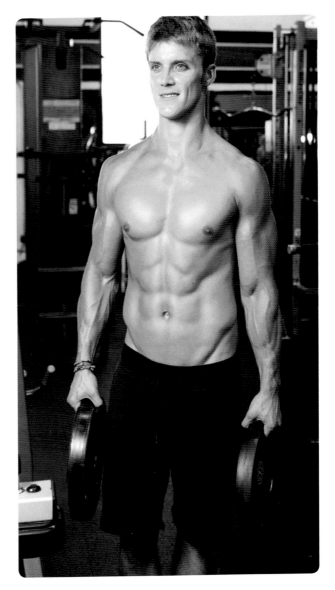

6. **Limit extraneous activities.** Keep in mind the fast tempo at which the ectomorph's metabolism beats. Your efforts here are to make quality weight stick, so it is important to limit both aerobic activity and long-term intense exercise efforts that can further stimulate an already raging metabolism. This extra work can cut into both your recuperation and, ultimately, further muscular gains. For example, performing an intense leg workout and then playing a strenuous game of basketball is counterproductive because the muscles that have been broken down through resistance training have not had ample time and nutrients to repair. The result will be a constant state of disrepair and no further gains.

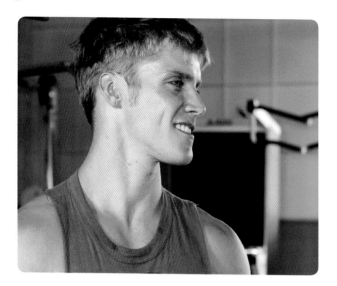

PHASE 1
WEEKS 1–4

MONDAY	Chest/Back/ Abdominals + 20-minute cardio
TUESDAY	OFF
WEDNESDAY	Legs
THURSDAY	OFF
FRIDAY	Shoulders/Arms/ Abdominals + 20-minute cardio
SATURDAY	OFF
SUNDAY	OFF

DEFINING THE PROGRAM

This book is broken down into three phases of progressive change, each lasting 4 weeks for a 12-week transformation that will result in noticeable improvements. During each phase, your workouts will target each body part/muscle group once per week. If you are able to train a particular muscle more than once per week, then that initial session was less than an all-out effort; there was something left in the tank. Here's an example: If you were playing baseball and made multiple trips up to the batter's box, you might not give your all each time, saving a little something for future at-bats. But if you approached the plate just once a week in an effort to go beyond where you've hit the ball previously, then you're programming your mind and body to go beyond your limits. The same holds true if you strive to lift more weight or perform an extra repetition—this is where the stimulation for growth truly happens.

The workouts are targeted and laid out for you, and the reliance on cardiovascular work is minimal (to maximize an anabolic or muscle-building state), so you may find that getting in all the meals is the most difficult part of the program. Building muscle tissue takes fuel and time, along with the proper training stimulus and recuperation. But even if you're not a foodie, don't fret. As your strength and output increases, so too will your appetite—to the point that you will soon look forward to your next meal. Keep in mind, too, that when you're not particularly hungry it is always easier to drink calories than it is to eat them. So if need be, drink a high-quality "weight gainer" shake (recipe contained herein) to keep your muscles fueled for performance and, ultimately, growth.

BEGINNER TRAINING PROTOCOL

The initial phase of training is less about the progression of weight and strength and more about firing from the working muscles, as well as feeling how muscles work together. For example, you'll feel your back muscles working with your chest during the descent portion of a bench press as your chest muscles firing during the ascent, yet both sets of muscles are working together to complete the movement. In this first phase you are looking at three days of weight training and four days off to maximize recuperation. Remember, more is not better. Better is better. A hint of abdominal and cardiovascular work is included. Myofascial rolling is also included before the workouts and stretching at the completion of your weight training for maximum usage and placement benefit.

PHASE 2
WEEKS 5–8

MONDAY	Back/abdominals + 20-minute cardio
TUESDAY	Chest/Biceps
WEDNESDAY	OFF
THURSDAY	Legs + 20-minute cardio
FRIDAY	Shoulders/Triceps/ Abdominals + 20-minute cardio
SATURDAY	OFF
SUNDAY	OFF

INTERMEDIATE TRAINING PROTOCOL

Now that you're firing from the correct muscles and confident with the program sequencing, you are ready to focus on increased power and lean muscle mass. You will add a fourth day of weight training in order to give more attention to all muscle groups and thoroughly exhaust them once per week—as well as attack them with the addition of a few new and different angles. Aside from maximal tension on the working muscles and less from ancillary muscles, your foremost goal is now building increased strength. For example, if your previous best was lifting 50-pound dumbbells for 6 reps on the incline press, your goal should be to get to 8 and then onward to the 55-pound dumbbells. Week in and week out, you won't always hit a new record, but you must try for records. And remember to keep it honest: write it down in your training diary (more on this later) only if the lift was done properly, with a full range of motion and absolute integrity.

PHASE 3
WEEKS 9–12

MONDAY	Back/Abdominals + 20-minute cardio
TUESDAY	Chest/Biceps/ Abdominals
WEDNESDAY	OFF
THURSDAY	Legs + 20-minute cardio
FRIDAY	Shoulders/Triceps/ Abdominals + 20-minute cardio
SATURDAY	OFF
SUNDAY	OFF

ADVANCED TRAINING PROTOCOL

The final, advanced phase of transformation is very similar to Phase 2 with the exception of additional and, sometimes, substitute or alternate exercises, as well as an extra day of cardio and abdominals to further help process and assimilate nutrients. Again, you are after record lifts that are honest in execution and, by now, the training, nutritional, and recuperation demands should be second nature. Regarding exercise, stick primarily with the basics, as they will never fail you and are your mainstay foundation toward building a 3-D physique. Stay true to them and, one day, your size M shirt will, by way of necessity, become L and onward and upward.

MYTH DEBUNKING AND TRUISMS

Like any undertaking, course, or challenge, there exist truths. Knowing not just the "what" but also the "why" is essential in understanding your unique ectomorphic body and how you will ultimately arrive at your goals. In any field, to accrue results, there are myths that must be refuted, for believing these myths will be counterproductive to your growth and development.

DEFINING TRUTH

Doubts need to be placed to rest, for wherever there are existing muscle cells, muscle can be built. I was forever made a believer years ago by that friend in high school. And while we can't change the shape of a muscle or our bone structure, we largely have control over its size and composition. Take for example a person born with high calf insertions or short biceps. Although he can't pull down or lengthen the calf or biceps, he absolutely can make them bigger. Although genetically ectomorphs tend to display narrow shoulders, additional width can be added by working on bringing out the medial or side head of the deltoids through various presses and laterals, as well as further widening the latissimus dorsi through varying versions of pull-downs and pull-ups. It's not about what we don't have, but rather defining what it is you have to work with and building from there.

DEFINING SELF-TRUTH

Scores of ectomorphs take up the quest for larger muscles only to quickly abandon it when they don't see immediate results. Of course they failed—after all, it takes not just a plan but also the consistent execution of a plan to make any gains. For the ectomorph especially, it would also seem to take considerable long-term effort to make any improvement at all. Still, many ectomorphs are the victims of self-sabotage, thwarting their own efforts to build muscle.

Recently, I had the pleasure of working with an ectomorph who had tried nearly everything in his quest to fill out and add more size. Still, despite his failure so far, he came to me hopeful, not hopeless. One of the first things I asked him was about his daily dietary intake. His reply was detailed and not the usual answer of "I am eating everything." Those struggling to gain weight tend to think they are eating enough, but usually upon closer inspection, they are eating an abundance of processed foods and sugar (energy), hardly the muscle-building nutrients we need for growth.

As I pressed on for exactly what he was eating, he mentioned meals like egg-white omelets. It became clear that the one thing absent in his diet was fats. His protein and carbs (especially his carbs) were high, but his lack of "good" fats was the largest dietary mistake holding him back. I explained that someone of his build and genetic predisposition had no business consuming just an egg-white omelet, from which, at best, he is only getting trace amounts of fat. He needed fat sources that include the yolks on a consistent basis. Not fat sources like pizza, sausage, or hot dogs, which contain saturated fats, but sources that would supply his body with unsaturated fats, such as almonds, avocados, olive oil, and salmon. I explained that the fats are what keep his muscles full and strong and slow down digestion from an already raging metabolism. Fats are also what satiate us and allow us to remain in

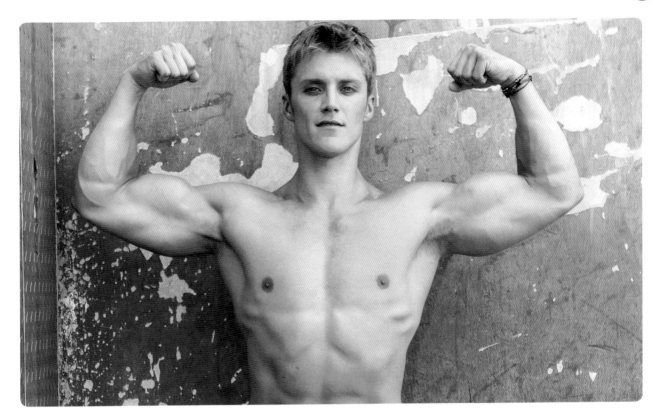

a positive nitrogen balance, or state in which there is a constant supply of protein available in the blood sugar and therefore yielding an anabolic or muscle-building state. Now, months later, he is at least 12 pounds bigger and just as lean as when we began.

For him, defining self-truth was taking a hard look at his diet, figuring out where he had gone wrong and then correcting it. You can do the same by examining what pertains to you and your unique gifts.

MYTH VERSUS TRUTH

We all have ideas about what is "true," but too often those truisms hold us back. Here are a few common self-sabotaging myths that you must put aside in order to see success.

• **Myth:** I am stuck this way.

• **Truth:** You are never stuck in any situation. Just think of Batman—he always finds a way out of situations—and you can, too. There may not be an easy or quick fix, but there is always a way to improve. Today we live in a very fast world in which many want it now. Give your fitness program time and a real go, and I promise you will put muscle on your body and be well on your way toward filling out that T-shirt. All you essentially need is a vision, plan, belief, fuel, progressive resistance training, and time, and you will grow. In the end, it's always You vs. You.

• **Myth:** Out of sight, out of mind. I'll just stay covered up and avoid the embarrassment.

• **Truth:** Always expose the muscle group you are training that day. This way you can see your muscles contracting as you are working them out. No matter how slight your build, how can you expect to improve your physique if you can't see it? When Arnold Schwarzenegger first came to the United States in the late 1960s, he was very impressive. He was big, a little soft, but developed everywhere—except his calves. And what did he do? He cut the lower portion of his jeans to expose his then very weak lower legs. And through a never-quit attitude, he ultimately built a pair of calves that were the equivalent in standout size to his superlative chest and amazing biceps. The lesson here? Expose the weak so that it may become strong. A word of caution: Avoid wearing extremely form-fitting compression gear, as this is the other end of the spectrum. Just wear comfortable clothes to the gym, clothes you can both breathe and work out in that also allow you to see the muscles you are training.

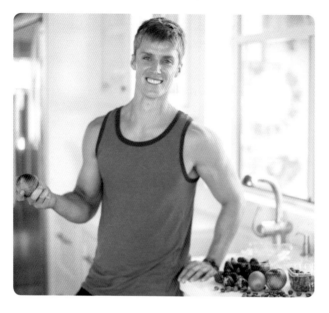

first time around. Get in, lift more weight in good form or best a previous "record," feed the muscle and recover, and you will improve.

• **Myth:** I'll just keep refining. I don't really want to build.

• **Truth:** Please stop right now. Stop this perpetual untruth. You can't possibly paint and furnish a house until the walls are built. You cannot refine something if there is nothing to refine. The word *refinement* is often just used in weight training as an excuse to put off the hard work of building.

• **Myth:** I'll just be good at multiple things.

• **Truth:** You could certainly perform well on both the field and in the gym, but these are two completely different modalities. Running is great cardio exercise, but it is too strenuous recuperative-wise for the hardgaining ectomorph who seeks to put weight on, not take it off. Ectomorphs should avoid strenuous cardio but keep some semblance of it in their training (more on this later). For example, ride the bike instead of running, which is less likely to interfere with your legs' recuperation from weight training. My advice: pick a road and stick with it. If you veer off the path, you risk getting lost in ways that lead to a new destination—and not the one you were aiming for. Bigger or faster—choose your destiny, and stick with it!

THE PRINCIPLES OF THE GAME

I've never been a fan of rules or "this must be done" commandments. We are not dealing in absolutes, but rather the always-in-flux human body. You want to grow new tissue and, ultimately, change your body's composition. Sure, everyone is unique, especially ectomorphs, but I do believe in principles that say, "This has worked for others, and I can find a way to make it work best for me." The following principles are the hardgainer seedlings that will over time grow the practitioner into a powerhouse tree.

• **Myth:** I have no appetite and can't possibly eat all that food. Besides, the body can only process like 25 grams of protein per meal.

• **Truth:** First, while it is true that any excess of calories consumed above normal body maintenance and activity level—be they in the form of protein, carbs or fats—can be stored as body fat, chances are that the ectomorph's speedy metabolism will more than likely burn off those extra calories. And second, the nutritional protocol outlined in this book does not call for bottomless plates and forced or binge eating. You are not required to wake up at some early-morning hour to down a protein shake or steak. In addition, the more muscle mass you carry, the more protein you will both require and assimilate. Be assured that someone who weighs 230 muscular pounds is taking in and can utilize more protein per meal than a 165-pounder. As your workload increases, your appetite will increase to follow suit. And as mentioned previously, you can always drink calories when you're not very hungry, as opposed to eating them. *Bon appétit!*

• **Myth:** The more times I work a muscle per week, the more growth I can stimulate.

• **Truth:** The more times you work a muscle per week, the more overtrained it will be, resulting in not only a lack of muscle stimulation but also possible injury. In exercise, more isn't better—smarter is better. If you are able to train a particular muscle more than once per week, then you didn't sufficiently train the muscle the

Target set. This is the training stimulus from which muscle growth starts and ultimately occurs. If a muscle is not subjected to a progressively heavier load, then it will not grow. One might "fool" the body with a new or different workout or some such muscle confusion, but at the end of the day if you've not lifted more or improved in some measured step, new muscle growth will not occur. Aside from warm-up sets or all-out sets, target sets are the key to increased performance and bigger muscles. And they need to be kept honest and with integrity, progressively heavier in both poundage and repetitions achieved and ultimately, recorded in your training journal (more on this later).

Tension on the muscle. This is a huge factor in muscle growth and yet is often overlooked. There's little point in bench pressing a heavy weight if it takes a severe arching of the back or shortened range of motion, or curling a barbell using more lower back than biceps just to say you lifted a certain amount of weight. Although placing tension on a given muscle usually results in lifting less weight overall, the results are well worth it. Because most of us are programmed to complete a set at all costs, form can go out the window rather quickly—which defeats the purpose of why we are in the gym to begin with. Ask yourself one question: Are you into bodybuilding (developing muscle mass) or powerlifting (lifting the most weight)? If quality real-world solid muscle is your desire, then your answer should be "bodybuilding."

Rest. Always rest as long as is necessary between sets to be able to give your all to your next target set. You're in the gym to increase your lean muscle mass, not to shave time off your workouts as other athletes may strive to do. Certainly recovery from a set of squats will require more time than, say, a set of lateral raises. Rest time is instinctive. Ignore the clock or a countdown until the next set but instead, rely on an internal beat that says "I'm ready to go." Ask yourself how much time is needed in order to do your last set the correct way, and then proceed.

Advanced techniques. There have been dozens of techniques developed over the years to increase intensity. Everything from muscle confusion (changing your workouts) to triple drop sets (training beyond normal muscle failure within a given set). They all have merit, but the rest/pause technique is my favorite for increasing muscle mass. This technique calls for you to perform a given number of repetitions until temporary muscle failure, then rack the weight, rest a few seconds, and perform another one to two repetitions beyond what you might normally be able to do. This serves multiple purposes. It allows you to spot yourself should you run into trouble during your set, it allows you to train beyond your normal threshold and establish new records, it allows you to keep the tension where it belongs and, above all, it allows you to build new muscle tissue.

The art of the rep. Theories exist regarding the time allocated between sets. Slow, fast, multisecond count . . . and ad infinitum. Each rep consists of a negative, or lengthening of the muscle (for example, the downward extension during a barbell curl), followed by the positive (the upward flexion or shortening portion of the curl), and then the static or contracted position. The greatest amount of muscle breakdown (stimulus for growth) occurs during the negative phase, and so it is crucial to achieve a full range of motion to fully develop a muscle. Use a controlled lowering, as if pulling back an arrow while setting up a shot on a bow, and an explosive positive, as if firing the arrow. Avoid very slow repetitions, as this will restrict the amount of weight employed and therefore interfere with muscular gains. Above all, always be in total control of each repetition, and use a weight that you are able to handle. Run with intelligence, not ego.

Prioritization. In any endeavor, most people begin with their strengths, not their weaknesses. In countless gyms across the globe, come Monday, men will train their chests and biceps. Why? These are the "showboat" muscles—most guys have decently built chests and biceps. But most men usually also display glaring weaknesses, such as lack of back development or the "light-bulb physique," in which a good upper body sits essentially on stilts. Prioritize, and be honest with yourself in what is lacking. Begin the week when you are strongest mentally and physically, and attack those lagging body parts with a passion. As an ectomorph, work on overall thickness. Exercises like side laterals and concentration curls, generally termed "finishing exercises", must take a backseat to bread and butter movements such as deadlifts and rows, which are the true mass builders.

Better yourself. If you've ever been to a bodybuilding show, at first glance it might seem odd. Oiled and tanned "athletes" in basically their underwear posing in front of hundreds or thousands of people. Where's the appeal? Well, for the competitors— aside from a smörgåsbord of cheat meals once the competition is over—the true motivation and reward is in besting their previous best. Each individual has no control over how the other participants look come the day of the show; only making sure they look their absolute best. Adopt this mentality: look better than your previous form, and you've won. That's what this whole endeavor is about—improvement and the ongoing pursuit of personal advancement. Your job and main focus should be in besting last year's model of you.

THE MENTAL EDGE

Overcoming obstacles all comes down to heart. It's not about genetics or gifts or limitations—you can overcome nearly any obstacle if you just believe you can. But before you see changes to the physical, you must reprogram yourself mentally. Develop a mental edge—then and only then will you proceed with confident progressions.

In developing a fitness plan for the hardgainer, "OK" comes from interest, "good" comes from desire, and "great" comes from obsession. And in order for you, the ectomorph, to succeed, you must be obsessed with a plan. You are attempting to overcome a major obstacle—your own raging metabolism—and to do that you must play by your own set of rules. The approach is definitely not "lift as much as you can and eat until sick," but instead a breaking through of previously set limits, both mental and physical. Prior to any plan and its execution, preparing the mind makes all the difference. Before any transformation, one must first process the journey.

If you've picked up this book, chances are you've come to terms with, accepted, and now demand that you, the ectomorph, need more. You've accepted the challenge that you can work toward more and, above all, that it's possible, knowing that hard, consistent work yields results. Goals are most obtainable via a linear path. And it starts with questioning your process: Are you laterally or linearly advancing?

Although the image of being "skinny" or underweight may be deeply burned into the recesses of your brain, you have to be willing to see past who you were and are, and focus on who you want to be and who you will become. Banish the thought of being undersized and scrawny, and imagine being full and muscular. It has always helped me to put a picture on my fridge door of someone whose physique I wish to emulate, so I would have no choice but to see it daily. It becomes a reminder of why I am lifting these heavy weights and eating all these chicken breasts in the first place.

One of the greatest lessons that I ever took to heart on programming the mind for success came from an up-and-coming bodybuilder. As one of the favorites and front runners going into the contest, he was asked if he could indeed be the best in the world. He replied, "Someone has to be the best in the world," and then followed with a question of his own: "Why not me?" Initially, it seemed overwhelmingly absurd for him to think of himself as the number one in the world. But ultimately, his question made it concretely clear that he had the necessary mental edge. Once the thought of being the world's best became tangible in his mind, the physical act of being crowned became his reality—and may have been actually less taxing than the mental work he had done prior to his first of many wins. That man would become a six-time Mr. Olympia.

The ectomorph's journey is an exciting one because it is a private war. Unlike a Mr. Olympia, you don't have to convince others of your greatness or potential, just yourself. And once you do, a world of possibilities opens up. You need not rely on other players on the team performing optimally, because there are no other players, just you.

Somewhere along the way you may have bought into what you were fed all your life. You were labeled "thin," "skinny," "small," and a myriad of other negative adjectives. And, most probably, that is how you came to view yourself. And it is now up to you to break free of those false labels and to set about changing you for the better and progressively looking how you want to look. And most important, being who you wish to be. Believe that there are no limits.

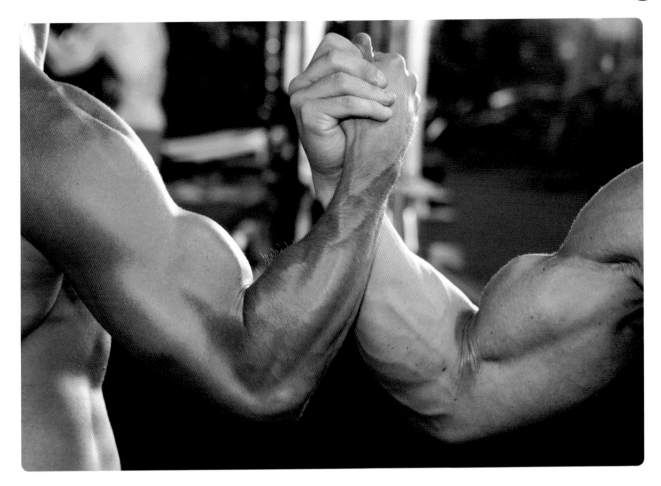

FREEING YOUR MENTAL LIMITS

As you familiarize yourself with this book, you'll be further able to visualize what the "new and improved" you will look like. Read the words and study the photos, which will help for clarity. Work on seeing yourself in the photos doing the work and attaining results. These visions are the pillars that will hold up the foundation of your success.

Visualization is a highly powerful tool. You must first "see" who you want to become and then project that image outward. For your endeavors here, that translates to lifting heavier poundages than previously hoisted, eating the required meals to nourish your body, and resting to repair muscle tissue. If you can see it, you can achieve it. Think of it as building a train track. Although not every day results in laying down a new piece of track, over time, a consistent laying down of a piece of track here and there will eventually help to ensure that the train will run.

The only difference between a skinny hardgainer and a heavily-muscular one is in the execution of planned action. In other words, an actual concrete, physical progressive undertaking to replicate your ultimate vision and win clear mental mastery over your goals.

Mental mastery is not some unknown secret or rare commodity. It's something we all have the power to harness at will. We can choose to use it or allow it to use us. And since we all have self-doubt from time to time, it's about forging ahead through those clouded moments. For every bodybuilding show or photo shoot, I began with a clear picture in my head of how I wanted to look, and I did everything within my power to achieve or surpass that look come the day of the event. It wasn't magic. I simply carried on day in and day out to the best of my ability and, slowly but surely, my body followed suit and made the desirable changes to eventually catch up with my mind. I was never in a rush because I knew it would take time to achieve my goals. Instant gratification and results do not complement each other nearly as well as consistency and true results.

It never mattered to me who else was competing, because I had zero control over how others looked—only how I looked. Knowing that there are few things in life we have control over other than our bodies is a powerful truth. So why not channel all that positive energy into bettering yourself?

FEAR NOT FAILURE

For many, the fear of possibly failing is too often a strong indicator of an unwillingness to even begin. If your fear of failure is greater than your will to succeed, you will not achieve. Failure doesn't scare me, for at best it's temporary. What scares me is the possibility of being ill-prepared for something I am passionate about, and I do everything I can to ensure victory.

A lot of times we either consciously or subconsciously bring our own progression to a screeching halt. It would seem as if when positive change occurs, we self-sabotage—perhaps thinking we don't deserve for things to be this good. But guess what? You do deserve all the good things, so get out of your own way, for self-derailment is a dream stopper. If you hear a voice in your head that says *you can't do something,* ignore it. Only you have the power to thwart or to empower yourself. No one else has this control over you. And since it is indeed you in the driver's seat, it is up to you to decide in which direction you will go. Remember, good things come to those who take action!

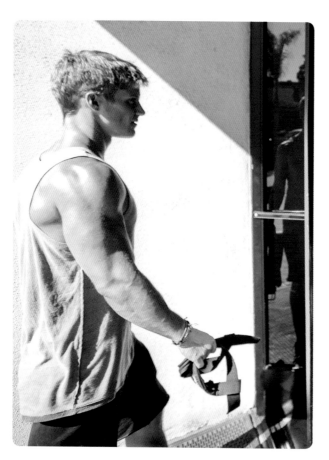

THE MENTAL ARSENAL

There are several key elements that you must pack in your mental arsenal. Visualize these important elements, and then take action.

A new level. The strongest weapon in your arsenal is the will to surpass your previous best in any fitness endeavor. Ask yourself, "What noticeable improvements have I made?" Push yourself beyond your previous bests, which can keep you motivated for oodles of time. Here's what's great about what we do in the gym: you can't buy it, you have to earn it, and then it's yours.

Architect of aggression. As adults, in most instances, certainly most public ones, we must keep aggression in check. In the gym, though, all bets are off. This is the one venue in which you don't have to keep it in check. You are here to construct You Version 2.0. Fuel up with quality muscle-building foods, take your pre-workout supplement, crank that music up, and clench your weightlifting belt in hand. Who wouldn't want to take advantage of going to war with a stacked arsenal with only the thought of victory? Perhaps be mindful of others and your surrounding space, and never mistake dropping or throwing weights for intensity.

Fat Lady Sings. Bettering yourself and having others recognize it is a form of motivation, provided your motivation is largely for yourself and not just for the approval of others. Stay humble. Fight the urge to be cynical: instead of putting down the other guy, put up yourself. We all share the ability to disallow others' negativity to adversely affect our positive actions. Manage your own madness by excelling and do not listen to others saying "you can't," when the literal translation is them saying "they can't." No one—and I mean no one—has control over you or the right to limit what you may become. The show goes on until you say so. Remember that the naysayers are either unable or unwilling to attempt to become what you are. Let your actions define your character, and unveil your new body on your own terms.

Purpose. While many start out strong at the beginning of a journey, few complete the mission unscathed, and even fewer complete it at all. Remember why you started this journey, keeping one foot in front of the other. It's about pursuant offense, not worrisome defense. Remember that your efforts are enough and that they are worth it. Suffering is temporary, results are eternal.

Now I can see. Training without a clear plan that you can see will at best result in one step forward, two steps back. Sticking to a concrete plan makes all the difference toward getting you to your goals. Visualize your goal and then formulate a clear plan. And don't be in a rush to get started; be committed to get started.

Make technology work for you. This is the digital age and there is no better time for you to act than now. With all of the advances in training, nutrition, and supplementation, nearly all of the guesswork has been taken out of designing a plan that fits you and your unique needs. And the portability of electronics today means you can carry your routine, diet, and even this book with you at all times for immediate and easy reference. Use every tool to your advantage!

Define yourself. Only you can define you. Only you can set your limits. You are free to be who you want to be, and if that equates to a better you, bring it on. If you truly wish to reap the most of your genetics, you have to be willing to go to war with yourself, but not against yourself. In other words, ask yourself, how am I getting in my own way? What stops me from crossing over the threshold to success? Once you have those answers, you can reprogram your mind for victory.

Self-affirmation. Of course you're excited. Of course you're excited to begin, and even more excited for results. It is the affirmation from within, not the daily selfies posted on social media with a hundred "Likes," that leaves you with a good sense of self and internal justification for continuing your battle. It's truly not about the final destination, but about today and about knowing that you are doing good work, consistently. Self-affirmation comes from besting a previous record in the gym (target set), putting on a shirt that fits snugly around your arms, or a glance in the mirror that shows improvement.

Passion over destiny. The outcome lies not in the cards, but rather in your hands. You and you alone are the author of your own destiny. It is you who ducks under the squat bar when the gym is empty because it's a holiday. It is you who scarfs down meal 4 when you're not even hungry, knowing that meal 5 is just around the corner. And it is you who can proudly look into the mirror knowing that you are the one behind your success. Passion, not destiny, is what keeps you going when you have the desire and heart to continue on, but not necessarily the reserves.

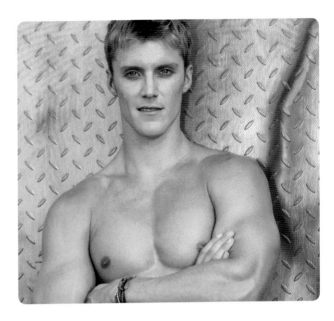

THE TAKEAWAY

Motivation cannot be coerced or forced. It can come from a variety of sources, no matter how minute they may seem. Sometimes it comes in spurts. In the course of one week, I had a book released, a new weight-lifting belt arrive with my name on it, and a new supplement delivered that I was eager to try. Individually, any of the three were cause for motivation, but all three made me feel supercharged!

It need not matter how you got it—just the fact that you did. Some of us are internally motivated, others need a trainer, cause, or gun to the head to get it together. But once you've found your motivation, hold on to it.

Gaining, retaining, and utilizing the mental edge is an ongoing process, a sword that must be continually sharpened. Just as every meal and repetition brings you closer to your goals, the thought behind the muscle must be present like oxygen to the brain.

Not every attempt succeeds; what matters most is that you try. Keep moving forward. Only you can set and reach your destination, and that in and of itself is very exciting. Do not reverse yourself and switch gears, such as working on building muscle mass one week and then concentrating on "refining" the next. Do not second-guess yourself. Do not listen to the first person who gives you advice. Do not even look at others who may be more genetically gifted. Do not abandon the journey until you reach your destination. As the old saying goes, "Slow and steady wins the race." You can and will overcome certain genetic limitations (which everyone possesses) provided you stay the course.

EATING FOR GROWTH

Just face it—the majority of diet books out there are not designed with you in mind. The general populace is looking to lose weight (in whatever form that may be) as quickly, effortlessly, and painlessly as possible. But a book that covers gaining weight? To many, it would be like putting true crime in the children's section. But you, the ectomorph, are a different breed.

The ectomorph has but one mission: to increase his body weight and, specifically, lean muscle mass. You are not looking to slim down and fit into jeans or aspiring to fasten the top button of a dress shirt. You are looking to break through previous dimensions—and shirts—and to do that, you have to pay special attention to not just the barbell plate, but also to your dinner plate.

BUILDING A BIGGER, BETTER YOU

You'll often hear that nutrition alone is 90 percent of your results. But to suggest this is to suggest that to eat correctly will yield the same 90 percent of results. That would be terrific, but it is tantamount to collecting thousands of auto parts and expecting the car to be able to run without being constructed. You also need a mechanic to correctly build that car, or in this case, exercise and recuperation to correctly build your bigger body. Equal structured parts composed of workout, recuperation, and nutrition replicated over time is what will build the new and improved you.

The ectomorphic metabolism is generally efficient at burning body fat, so it's safe to assume that you have some semblance of abdominal definition on your midriff. Even if you don't, the program outlined in this book will simultaneously build and harden your physique. But you absolutely *must* eat correctly. For your body type, skipping breakfast or consuming just an egg white omelet at the complete expense of the all-important yolks or not having carbs after early afternoon—or any number of counterproductive and outdated dietary misgivings—will not bring you closer to your physique goals and only further serve to frustrate you.

Weight gain, however, doesn't mean eating near limitless foods and packing on sloppy pounds. Not only is this unhealthy, but it also does little in the way of enhancing your body's aesthetics. The goal is adding quality muscle, and that cannot be rushed, most especially with the ectomorph. For example, if you aim to add 2 pounds of muscle per month, that's 24 pounds of muscle in one year. That is a tremendous amount of muscle! Quality, not quantity.

Overcoming or conquering the calorie-burning ectomorphic metabolism is not about overloading or stuffing your belly, but instead it is about consistency and, believe it or not, some leniency. The rapid ectomorphic metabolic rate has a tendency to break down food and not store it as body fat, so you need not adhere to a strict diet regimen of dry chicken breasts with no sauce and plain baked potatoes with no butter. Some of the added fats commonly served with these foods are actually beneficial to you because they will slow down the rate of digestion and help to bind foods, or have calories "stick" to you and will ultimately yield larger muscles.

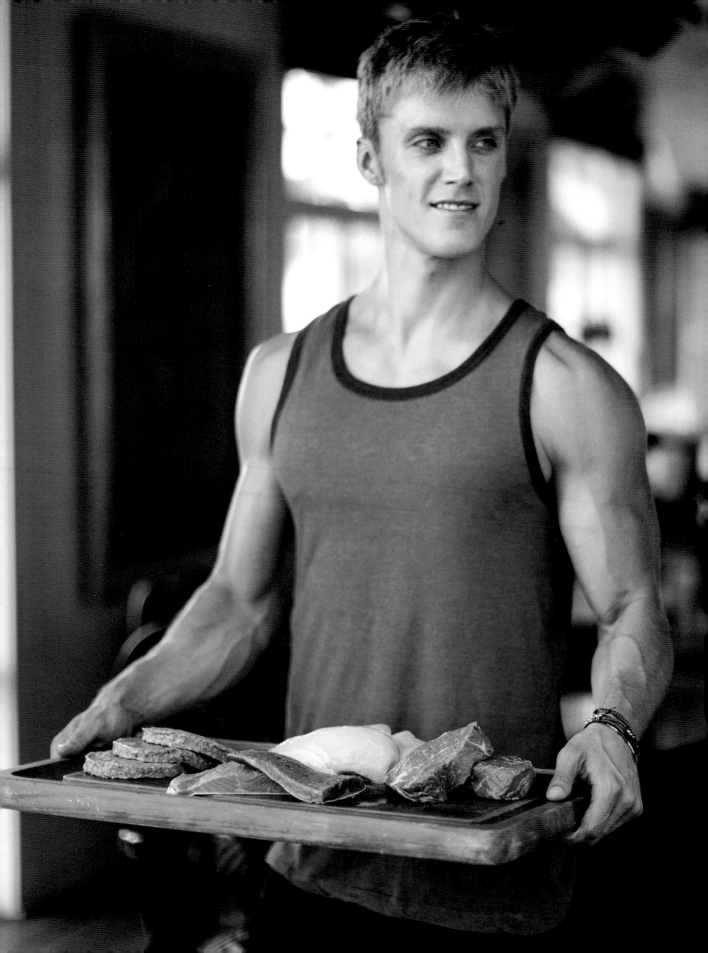

This doesn't mean a diet of cookies and cakes, which in the end are just energy and contain, at best, trace amounts of protein. What this does mean is a back-to-the-basics, meat-and-potatoes nutritional plan that augments your training and recuperation. These three things combined will truly build the hardgainer.

You are erecting a structure, as opposed to whittling it down, and you therefore require more raw materials. What is an advantage over those trying to lose weight is that your intake calls for a consistent surplus of nutrients. And along with the consistency in the proper nutrients is consistency in the frequency of those nutrients. You can't skip meals. The speed at which the ectomorph's metabolism runs means that too many missed meals can quickly lead to cannibalization of precious muscle tissue.

You probably have some understanding of basic nutrition, but perhaps less about how to apply it to the ectomorph's unique needs. The text that follows is geared specifically to you, and it does not apply to those with differing body types and goals.

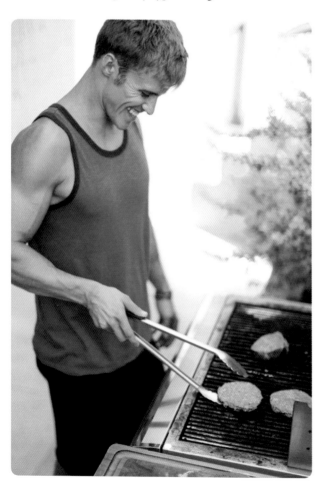

THE NUTRITIONAL ARMAMENT

Three macronutrients are largely responsible for both the amount and quality of muscle mass on your physique: proteins, fats, and carbohydrates. By having a proper understanding of each of these macronutrients, as well as learning how to manipulate and apply them, you will literally transform your body by adding muscle and losing body fat, simultaneously!

PROTEIN

Protein is essential for muscle growth and maintenance, helping to repair muscle tissue after muscle breakdown (exercise). You must consistently take in protein to promote an anabolic, or muscle-building, state.

Amino acids, which build muscle tissue and repair damaged tissues, are the building blocks of protein. Approximately 20 different amino acids make up the proteins in the human body. Nine of those (phenylalanine, valine, threonine, tryptophan, methionine, leucine, isoleucine, lysine, and histidine) are considered "essential." An essential amino acid (also known as an indispensable amino acid) cannot be synthesized by the body and therefore must be supplied by the foods in your diet.

For growth purposes, take in at least one gram of protein per pound of body weight—and even a bit extra to support new growth. For example, it is recommended that a male weighing 165 pounds takes in about 200 grams of protein per day, divided into four to six small meals.

You are probably reading this and thinking, "You want me to eat four to six meals every day? No way!"

I say, "Yes, way."

You will be able to eat that often for a few reasons. Sure, it will at first seem to be a struggle because you are not used to consuming that much protein daily, but as you become accustomed to eating more and are rigorous in keeping up with your training, your appetite will increase in order for you to push your body to new heights. Additionally, the meal plan to follow calls for three whole meals and two shakes daily, which decreases the actual food you must eat. Again, it is always easier to drink your calories than it is to eat them. Initially, you may need to increase that to three shakes daily and eat only two whole meals to better accommodate your (current) lesser appetite. Because whole food digests slower, as your appetite increases over time, it would better serve you to consume more whole food meals, which digest slower than protein powders, thusly keeping your muscles nourished, full, and primed for growth at all times.

FIRST-CLASS PROTEIN SOURCES

The following foods, generally animal sources, are complete in amino acids and have a high biological value (BV). That is, they are largely able to be digested by the body and are used for muscle growth and repair.

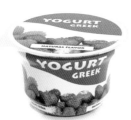

- Eggs
- Milk
- Cheese
- Yogurt
- Beef
- Chicken
- Turkey
- Fish
- Protein powder

SECOND-CLASS PROTEIN SOURCES

The following foods, which are from vegetable sources, work well with first-class protein sources by adding additional protein to your meals. They are by themselves, incomplete protein sources and must be combined with other foods to produce a complete essential amino acid profile.

- Nuts
- Beans
- Seeds
- Grains

WHOLE FOOD VS. SHAKES

Most, if not all, of your meals should come from whole food sources, which digest more slowly than protein powders; however, with the large amount of food necessary to properly fuel the ectomorph and to keep him in an anabolic state, along with the busy lifestyles we all maintain today, protein powder shakes are a very convenient way to help accommodate fuel demands.

The ideal ingestion of proteins would be to have a whole meal prior to your workout to allow for a slower and more sustained release of nutrients to hard-working muscles. Protein powders in easily assimilated and predigested shakes are best consumed post-workout, when there is an immediate need to replace lost nutrients and begin the muscle-repairing/building state. You need to consume protein—no matter what type—at every meal to stay in what is known as a "positive nitrogen balance," which is basically a state of muscular growth, or anabolism. There are generally four basic kinds of protein powders: whey, casein, egg albumin, and soy.

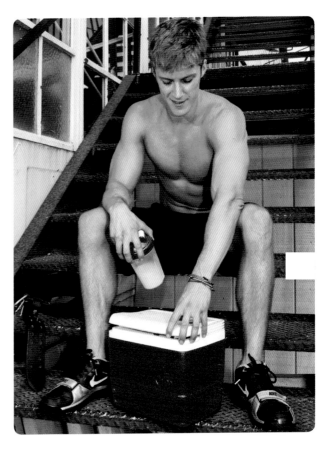

PROTEIN POWDERS

Whey protein, derived from cow's milk, has a very high BV that is rapidly absorbed and is considered a quick-release protein. It mixes easily and is best utilized immediately after training to begin the recuperative process.

Casein is considered a slower-release protein and is best utilized prior to bed for satiety and a slower rate of digestion. Casein, like whey, comes from cow's milk, but it is derived from the curds while whey is in the liquid portion. Though it has a lower BV than whey, it has a slower rate of digestion and will remain in the system for a longer period of time.

Egg albumin contains a very high BV and was the original standard of protein powder during the fledgling years of sports nutrition. It has been successfully used for decades, either before or after workouts for great results.

Soy is one of the few plant proteins that is considered a complete protein and can best be utilized as a meal replacement. One of its advantages over other protein powders is that it contains no lactose sugar, and those who are lactose intolerant can consume it with no worries.

FATS

Of at least equal importance to the ectomorph as protein, fats are essential to the further acquisition of lean tissue, as well as to normal body function. Skin and cell maintenance, the health of eyes and hair, lowering of cholesterol levels and disease prevention, are just some of the benefits of consuming the right kind of fats.

Concentrated sources of energy, fats clock in at a dense nine calories per gram. This is more than twice the number of calories in both protein and carbohydrates (four calories per gram). Fats can be further divided into subcategories including both saturated (bad fats) and unsaturated (good fats). The body doesn't digest saturated fats well and tends to deposit them where they can build up, while unsaturated fats are used for various bodily maintenance and optimal health.

For bodybuilding purposes, fats are vital in the fortifying of tissues and joints, which allows you to lift progressively heavier poundage and, ultimately, in having muscle "stick" to you. That is, overcoming a sometimes raging metabolism that continues to burn up calories and utilize stored energy for the building up of and keeping newly acquired muscle tissue.

UNSATURATED FATS (CONSUME WITH MODERATION)
- Avocado
- Flaxseed oil
- Safflower oil
- Salmon and trout
- Raw nuts

SATURATED FATS (LIMIT OR AVOID)
- Cheese
- Fatty meats
- Fries
- Pastries

As mentioned previously, when I began helping an ectomorph to build his body, I asked about his diet. Although he was consuming a lot of protein and carbohydrates, his fat intake was very low. The result was that he was tired and weak and looked thin or stringy. His muscles had a flat look to them, as if someone had forced the air out of a balloon. My very first instruction to him was to take in more unsaturated fats. Within two weeks, his strength skyrocketed and his physique took on a much fuller and harder appearance. Fats, they do your body good.

CARBOHYDRATES

Carbohydrates provide the energy that puts both protein and fats to use in yielding new muscle tissue. Like protein, carbs clock in at just four calories per gram. And also like protein, all carbs are not created equal. Carbs can be classified into two main categories: simple and complex. Simple carbs, such as sucrose, are the sugars that can be found in processed foods such as cakes and candy, as well as in more nutritious foods like fruits and vegetables. Complex carbs are generally considered unrefined or unprocessed (processed carbs often have nutrients taken out to make for a longer shelf life).

Upon ingestion, carbs immediately begin to break down into simple sugars; as they are further digested they are absorbed into the bloodstream, where they are known as glucose, which is basically the fuel your body needs to run efficiently. As blood sugar levels rise, your pancreas secretes the hormone insulin, which acts to allow glucose to enter into the body's cells to be used as energy. Simple carbs tend to speed along this process, giving you quick, short bursts of energy, whereas complex carbs provide more sustained energy. The key for the growing ectomorph is to consume a slow-digesting meal prior to your workout, followed by an easily assimilated protein and simple carb after to immediately begin the growth and repair process.

SIMPLE CARBOHYDRATES (POST-WORKOUT)
- Fruit
- Some vegetables
- White bread
- Milk

COMPLEX CARBOHYDRATES (ALL OTHER MEALS)
- Quinoa
- Oats
- Whole-wheat breads and pastas
- Brown rice
- Yams

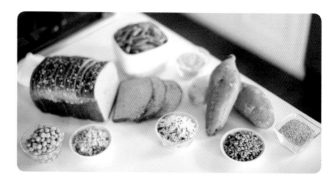

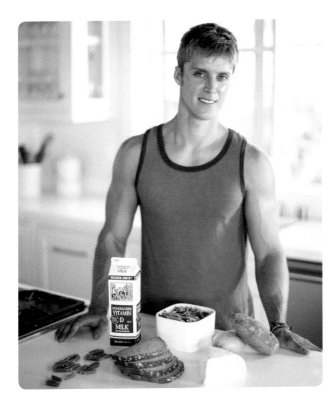

YOUR CALORIC NEEDS

To see results, you must also balance your caloric intake with your caloric expenditure—maximizing the former, while minimizing the latter. If you fail to take in enough calories, the furnace that is your metabolism will sacrifice muscle to fuel the body. If you overdo physical activity (excessive and/or strenuous cardio), then your body will be in a continual state of disrepair, and you risk losing weight.

Assuming our working ectomorph is 165 pounds, and most of that is lean muscle, he needs at least 165 grams of protein per day in order to maintain. Again, to put on weight, specifically muscle, you need to up that to about 200 grams daily. Fat intake, due to its dense caloric allotment and slower digestion, need only be about 100 grams daily.

Worth noting is that seven days per week, you must consume the necessary amounts of protein and fats to keep yourself in a continual and ongoing anabolic state. But carbs, your energy source, will fluctuate depending on your activity level, with the highest amounts ingested on workout days. So for rest days, aim for 200 grams, and double that to 400 on workout days.

Doing the math and putting it all together, you have: 200 x 4 = 800 calories from protein, 100 x 9 = 900 calories from fat and 400 x 4 = 1,600 calories from carbohydrates, equaling roughly 3,300 calories daily.

SAMPLE DAY

The following contains a sample training day's eating that provides roughly the type and quantity of nutrients you are looking for. Feel free to change the times and even sequence of the meals if it better suits you. Perhaps you prefer to train at 2:00 P.M., making meal 2 your pre-workout meal and meal 3 your post, so you would shift accordingly.

Note that meal 4 (the post-workout meal) contains only trace amounts of fat, while the other four contain at least 20 grams of fat. This is because the post-workout window is vitally important for repair and replenishment and the pre-digested whey, along with the simple sugars in the fruit and juice, allow for immediate nutrient absorption to allow the muscles to rapidly begin the growth and repair process, without being slowed down by high-calorie fats. (Note that this schedule works for me, but may not be for everyone. Make sure you get the proper amounts throughout your day, as the vitamins are more important than when you take them.)

Meal 1
8:00 a.m.
3 medium eggs
3 egg whites
¼ sliced avocado
2 slices whole-grain bread
1 cup oatmeal, cooked

Meal 2
11:00 a.m.
1½ scoops casein protein powder
2 tablespoons peanut butter
1 cup mixed berries
1 cup skim milk

Meal 3
2:00 p.m.
(pre-workout meal)
6 ounces cooked ground beef
4 ounces whole wheat pasta
broccoli (as much as you like)

Meal 4
5:00 p.m.
(post-workout meal)
1½ scoops whey protein powder
1 banana
1 glass of juice

Meal 5
8:00 p.m.
4 ounces cooked salmon
1 potato
1 salad

THE CHEAT MEAL

The cheat meal provides a temporary break from dieting, both mentally and physically. For the typical dieter, who wants to lose body fat, it is the chance to indulge in one big meal after a week of deprivation. In the case of the ectomorph, the cheat meal isn't about indulging in calories after limiting them, but instead eating favorite foods that may not be on the hardgainer's usual menu. A few cheat meals per week help keep body weight on and meet those caloric needs.

Even a cheat meal shouldn't be mindless indulgence, though. A less-than-ideal choice would be a stack of pancakes with butter for breakfast. There are, at best, trace amounts of protein in this meal, and the carbs and fats could keep you feeling full for hours, potentially forcing you to miss important meals. Additionally, the heavy carbs and fat will spike your energy levels and then quickly diminish, leaving you feeling tired and lethargic.

If you can, eat your cheat meal near the end of your day, particularly a training day when your body can use more fats for repair and growth. You could have perhaps a meatloaf as your last meal, which provides plenty of slow-digesting protein and fat. Carbs are optional—even encouraged—provided they do not make you too full to consume the crucial protein. The key is to take in the protein first, rather than filling up on carbs for energy that is just not needed for the low-expenditure of sleep.

THE PORTABLE KITCHEN

Training is the stimulus for muscular growth and development, but consistent efforts outside the gym (nutrition and recuperation) determine your physical composition. A little planning ahead will ensure that you cover your nutritional bases no matter where you are. Whether it be a flight, a movie, a class or the like, you can get quality nutrition when on the run and never derail your efforts or sacrifice your physique dreams.

Packing a zippered bag full of nuts, scooping protein powder into a shaker, and stacking previously prepared meals in plastic containers in a lunch box or cooler with an ice pack will help to guarantee that you get your meals in and keep within an anabolic state. Protein bars also offer a portable and convenient way to get those extra calories, and you can take them nearly anywhere.

With just a few ingredients and a portable blender you can whip up a powerful bodybuilding shake when on the go. Just combine 2 cups of whole milk or almond milk, 2 scoops protein powder, ½ cup dry oats, 1 banana, and a scoop of almond or peanut butter with some ice. Or blend it beforehand, snap on a travel lid, and drop it in your cooler.

You are rarely far from a meal these days. If you have no meals packed while you're on the road, you can always grab a burger. A meal need not be super clean for you and your unique needs, so if you desire that slice of cheese or bread, as long as you take in your quality first-class protein and opt to not skip meals later, indulge.

SUPPLEMENTATION

Supplements are just that—merely supplemental to food. Although they do make a difference to performance and, ultimately, muscle growth, opting for real muscle-building whole foods such as steak, potatoes, and greens over a protein shake provides you with slower-digesting nutrition any day. Having said that, with today's technology, there are some truly remarkable and effective supplements on the market that benefit the ectomorph.

Where once nutrition shelves were stocked with high-calorie shakes and powders that really only supplied an excess of sugar, today, you rarely see such items. Instead, ectomorphs who want to put on muscle will find shelves heavily stocked with quality protein powders, pre-workout mixes, fat-burners, and energy drinks. Competition is fierce and the consumer is more educated than ever. What we now know is that nutrient overloading, while important, must be balanced by equal parts consistency, quality training and recuperation.

The multibillion-dollar supplement industry is an enduring and thriving business in which many of the companies would have you regularly buying a vast array of "necessary" products. I'm here to tell you that you can build an incredible physique with or without supplements, and I repeat: supplements are merely supplemental to food. It is largely their ease of use, their portability and their ability to give you the choice to drink when you might not otherwise have the appetite to eat that make them so appealing.

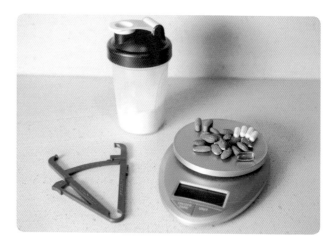

THE HARDGAINER'S HANDFUL

The following products will help to supplement you on the road to quality and consistent muscular gains. They have been listed by order of importance.

Multivitamin packets

These packets combine a variety of specific vitamins, minerals, fish oils, and other nutrients to give you targeted nutritional support for a variety of health and fitness needs. The commercials and media might have you believe that one pill taken daily will have it all. Not so for the hard-training athlete who requires even more nutrients than the average sedentary person. Vitamins and minerals supplement the macronutrient-dense foods typical of the bodybuilding diet. Multivitamin packets make the top of the list because they will ensure that everything is working efficiently internally to produce the desired external results.

Protein powders

The typical ectomorph faces the issue of getting in enough food, not only in the right amounts, but also in the necessary high quality. Protein powders are a portable, quick, and efficient way of taking in muscle-building and muscle-recovering protein and can be sipped instead of chewed. In the case of the ectomorph, consistently elevated protein levels are of paramount importance, so drinking protein shakes between whole meals is a great way to get that protein in and those numbers up. There are many blends on the market, including whey, casein, egg albumin, and soy, as previously covered.

Fish oils

Fish oil is a "good fat," that is, a fat that the body requires to function efficiently and properly. Fish oils are a great source of energy and supply antioxidant benefits. As such, they are highly beneficial to the heart as well as the tissue surrounding the joints and may reduce inflammation. The skin and hair also benefit from fish oil supplements. They are often included in multivitamin packets, and they are also sold separately.

Pre-workout supplements

This category of supplement is constantly reinventing itself while attempting to push the envelope. These supplements provide caffeine for energy and focus, nitric oxide for an increased muscle pump, creatine for fuller muscles, and other stimulants that help you power through your entire workout without waning. Containing very few calories, pre-workout supplements are meant to be used in conjunction with food for proper fueling. I love this category of supplement and perform nary a workout without them; they help to keep my intensity at high levels throughout and allow me to have a more focused and productive session. A word of caution: Some of these products are quite potent, so less is more. If you suffer from anxiety, hypertension, or other such conditions, avoid this category altogether. And it is recommended that pre-workout supplements be cycled, that is, not taken during an entire calendar year, because the body has a tendency to adapt to them.

Branched chain amino acids (BCAA)

BCAAs are the building blocks of protein, containing the three most important of the amino acids: leucine, isoleucine, and valine, which are responsible for protein synthesis (the process whereby individual muscle cells increase in size), energy production, and to prevent or decrease muscle breakdown. It is a good idea to take them first thing in the morning on an empty stomach in an effort to preserve muscle tissue, especially when having fasted through the evening.

Creatine

Creatine monohydrate increases the body's ability to produce energy rapidly, especially in the muscles. Creatine supplements, typically bought in flavored powders and mixed with liquid, increase intramuscular creatine stores and are perhaps the most widely used supplements in all of sports. Some users report strength increases as well as muscle fatigue resistance, while others report more fullness in their muscles and increased protein synthesis. Regardless, it is found mainly in red meat and has been shown to be less effective for endurance athletes but yields positive results for those engaged in bodybuilding-type training.

Glutamine

Glutamine is the most abundant amino acid found in the body and helps with repair and is responsible for protein synthesis, reducing muscle soreness and ultimately muscle growth. Athletes supplement with it directly after their workout to help with muscle repair and immune health.

Intra-workout supplements

These supplements, taken during a workout, are relatively new in the field. Sipped throughout training, they contain fast-acting carbohydrates, as well as essential amino acids directly responsible for helping muscle repair. The theory behind them is that because microdamage occurs to muscles while you work out and repair and growth occurs through nutrition and rest, taking a supplement during your workout will enhance performance, promoting increases in both muscle size and strength. As your workout progresses, your glycogen stores drop (the primary fuel muscles use for energy production). A good intra-workout supplement will provide new energy as well as help your muscles to repair when they are most receptive to nutrients.

ON DELIVERY SERVICES

If you are low on time, choices for delicious, nutritious meals that are big on taste and fuel can be delivered right to your door. You can supplement your own cooking with services like The Life Chef (www.lalifechef.com) that cook up delicious, high-quality foods.

TRY IT AT HOME

You can also try these recipes for yourself. They are easy, and take little time to prepare. (Recipes provided by The Life Chef at www.lalifechef.com).

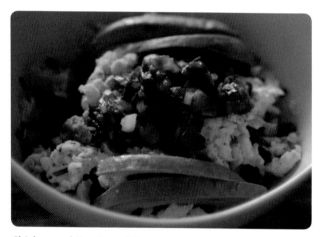

Chicken and Egg Scramble
Calories per serving: 679 / Fat: 12g / Carbs: 87g / Protein: 50g

CHICKEN AND EGG SCRAMBLE

SERVINGS: 1

- 3 small red potatoes
  (quarter and chop them into small pieces)
- 4 ounces cooked chicken breast
- 4 egg whites
- 2 tablespoons salsa or pico de gallo
- ½ avocado
- 1 teaspoon salt
- 1 teaspoon fresh ground pepper

DIRECTIONS:
Bring a skillet sprayed with nonstick spray to medium heat. Add chopped potatoes, and stir until they are hot and browned. Transfer to a medium bowl, and cover to keep warm.

Remove skillet from heat; clean, if needed. Re-spray skillet, and bring to medium heat. Add egg whites, chicken breast, salt, and pepper. Scramble until egg is fully cooked and chicken is warm. Stir in salsa, and transfer to the bowl of hash browns. Top with avocado.

TURKEY AND SPINACH EGG-WHITE SCRAMBLE WITH CINNAMON YAMS

SERVINGS: 2

- 4 ounces ground white-meat turkey
- 4 egg whites
- 1 Roma tomato
- 1 onion
- 1 garlic clove
- 1 medium zucchini, chopped small
- 1 teaspoon fresh ground pepper
- 1 teaspoon kosher salt
- 2 tablespoons olive oil
- 1 large yam
- ground cinnamon
- 1 tablespoon organic raw honey

DIRECTIONS:
Yams:
Preheat oven to 400°F.

Slice one large yam into ½-inch slices, and then place on baking sheet. Cook for approximately 20 minutes. Remove from oven, and drizzle honey over yams. Sprinkle with cinnamon to taste.

Scramble:
In a large pan, heat 2 tablespoon olive oil on medium heat. Add onion, and cook for 2 minutes. Add turkey meat, garlic, salt, and pepper, and cook until browned. Add tomato and zucchini, and cook for 3 to 4 minutes. Add eggs, and cook to desired consistency.

Serve with the yams.

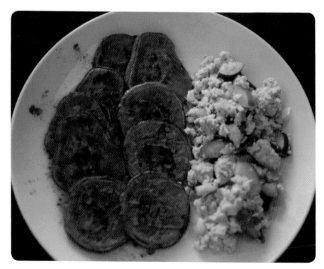

Turkey and Spinach Egg-White Scramble with Cinnamon Yams
Calories per serving: 631/ Fat: 29g / Carbs: 69 g / Protein: 47g

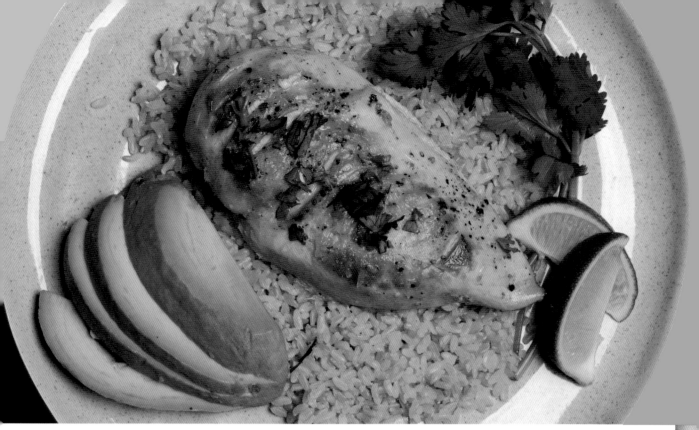

Cilantro Lime Chicken and Brown Rice *Calories per serving: 787 / Fat: 27g / Carbs: 81g / Protein: 55g*

SHAKE IT UP!

A protein-packed shake is perfect for the hardgainer. These recipes are both simple and effective. If a blender is unavailable, you can consume the ingredients individually.

Post-Workout Shake

Calories: 557 / Fat: 5 / Carbs: 85 / Protein: 43

2 medium bananas
1 tablespoons honey
1 cup low-fat milk (1–2%)*
1½ scoops whey protein isolate (chocolate or vanilla)

Blend all ingredients in a blender until thoroughly mixed.

*If water is desired instead of milk, use 2 scoops protein, and add an additional ½ tablespoon of honey.

Muscle Shake

Calories: 518 / Fat: 22 / Carbs: 42 / Protein: 38

1 cup milk or almond milk
1 scoop whey protein powder
1 cup frozen mixed berries (e.g., blueberries, raspberries)
¼ cup almonds or walnuts
  (peanut or almond butter may be substituted)

Place all ingredients in a blender, and blend for 30 seconds on high speed.

CILANTRO LIME CHICKEN AND BROWN RICE

SERVINGS: 2

2 eight-ounce boneless skinless chicken breasts
2 tablespoons coconut oil
3 tablespoons lime juice
¼ cup chopped cilantro
1 teaspoon garlic powder
1 teaspoon ground ginger
1 teaspoon chili powder
1 avocado
1 cup dry serving brown rice (about 2 cups cooked)
kosher salt and fresh ground pepper to taste

DIRECTIONS:

Rice:
Bring 2 cups of water to boil. Stir in rice, and reduce heat. Cover, and simmer for about 20 minutes. Remove from heat, and let stand for about 5 minutes.

Chicken:
In a medium skillet, warm coconut oil. Season chicken with salt and pepper, as well as the garlic powder, ground ginger, and chili powder, and add to skillet with lime juice. Cook about 6 minutes on each side or until the breasts are no longer pink in the middle.

Place 1 cup cooked rice on each of two plates, and top with chicken and juice from skillet. Garnish with chopped cilantro and sliced avocado.

ROASTED CHICKEN THIGHS WITH FINGERLING POTATOES AND BRUSSELS SPROUTS

SERVINGS: 2

6 chicken thighs (skin-on and bone-in)
4 cups fingerling potatoes
½ pound brussels sprouts (halved)
4 tablespoons olive oil
1 shallot, roughly chopped
2 tablespoons fresh rosemary, chopped
1 tablespoons fresh thyme, chopped
4 garlic cloves, sliced
1 lemon, thinly sliced
kosher salt and fresh ground pepper to taste

DIRECTIONS:

Preheat oven to 475°F.

In a large bowl, combine 2 tablespoons of the olive oil with the rosemary and thyme. Season with salt and pepper. Add chicken, and turn to coat.

On a rimmed baking sheet, toss potatoes, brussels sprouts, shallots, garlic, lemon, and remaining 2 tablespoons of olive oil; season with salt and pepper to taste. Spread out everything in an even layer, making sure that the chicken thighs are skin side up.

Roast about 22 to 25 minutes until brussels sprouts are tender, and the juices from the chicken run clear when pierced with knife.

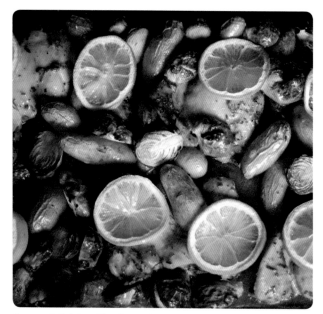

Roasted Chicken Thighs with Fingerling Potatoes and Brussels Sprouts
Calories per serving: 790 / Fat: 30g / Carbs: 70g / Protein: 60g

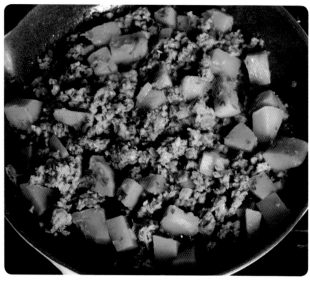

Italian Chicken Sausage and Butternut Squash Skillet
Calories per serving: 770 / Fat: 28g / Carbs: 80g / Protein: 45g

ITALIAN CHICKEN SAUSAGE AND BUTTERNUT SQUASH SKILLET

SERVINGS: 2

2 pounds fresh Italian chicken sausage (casing removed)
3 tablespoons fresh oregano, chopped
2 tablespoons Italian parsley, chopped
½ teaspoon black pepper
2 tablespoons olive oil
3 cups of 1-inch cubed butternut squash
5 garlic cloves
1 yellow onion, chopped
2 serrano peppers
½ teaspoon sea/kosher salt
½ cup organic chicken stock

DIRECTIONS:

Mix sausage, black pepper, Italian parsley and 1 tablespoon of the oregano in bowl. (Leave one tablespoon of oregano for the skillet.)

In a large lidded skillet or Dutch oven, heat olive oil over medium-high heat. Add sausage mixture, and with a large spoon or spatula, break mixture into large pieces, cooking until browned, about 6 to 7 minutes.

Add squash, garlic, onion, remaining oregano, and serrano peppers, along with salt and pepper to taste. Let cool, and stir vegetables until they begin to feel soft, about 3 minutes.

Add stock, and cover. Reduce heat to low-medium and simmer for about 20 minutes, stirring occasionally.

PAN SEARED TUNA WITH STEAMED BROCCOLI AND BAKED POTATO

SERVINGS: 1

6 ounces ahi tuna steak/fillet
1 large baked potato
1 cup broccoli, cut into bite-sized florets
2 tablespoons extra virgin olive oil
salt and pepper

DIRECTIONS:

Potatoes:
Preheat oven to 425°F.

Rub the potatoes with olive oil, sprinkle them with salt and pepper and then prick them with the tines of a fork. You can lay them directly on the oven rack or place them on a baking sheet. Cook them for 45 to 60 minutes, until their skin is crispy and sticking one with a fork meets no resistance.

Broccoli:
Place ¾ inch of water in a saucepan with a steamer, and bring to a boil. Add the broccoli and cover; reduce heat to medium, and steam just until tender, about 5 minutes.

Tuna:
Heat a medium-sized skillet to medium-high. Lightly brush both sides of tuna with olive oil. Lightly sprinkle sea/kosher salt and coarse ground black pepper on both sides. Place in skillet, and sear about 2 to 3 minutes on each side. (Cooking time depends on the thickness of the fish. Check side of tuna to see how fish is cooking. Meat will turn gray on sides as it heats.)

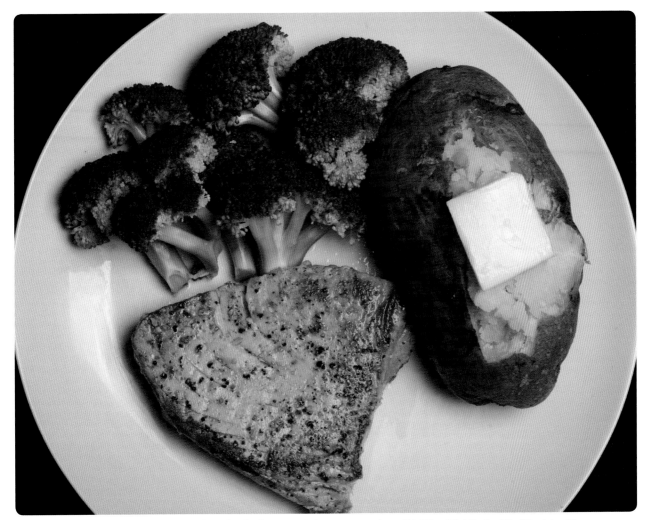

Pan Seared Tuna with Steamed Broccoli and Baked Potato *Calories per serving: 650 / Fat: 30 / Carbs: 70g / Protein: 50g*

NUTS, BOLTS, AND BARBELLS

We've all been there when a new item has arrived. Anxiously, you rip open the box, toss the instructions aside, and just grab the item in question. Sometimes you can figure it out on your own, but if you're like me, the instructions are a very necessary place to start—and not just for the "how" but also for the "why." This chapter contains action items or principles in motion—the essential instructions—that will allow you to get more out of your item, or in this case, your body.

THE TRAINING DIARY

Keeping an updated training diary is like having a physical representation of your brain on hand for instant access at all times. All the guesswork and theory is eliminated with a journal of your journey. How detailed and how often you update it is up to you and your abilities. At the very least, keeping a record of target sets, goals, your workouts, and your nutritional intake will track your progress and even tell you what is and what is not working. If you're willing to invest thousands of hours in the gym and at the dinner table in building your physique, then surely spending a few minutes recording vital data a few times per week is not a lot to ask.

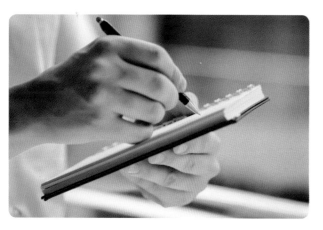

OLD VS. NEW

These workouts, although progressive, are raw by nature. One will be hard pressed to find the terms isolation, mobility, stabilization and the like applied to the ectomorph vocabulary—and for good reason: We are concerned with brute strength and size, not finesse and tranquility. We are here to rock your foundation. Words such as explosive, compound, and force are much more appropriate in terms of truly advancing the hardgainer. Within these pages, we are not after balancing on the ball or other such techniques, but rather repetitiously and explosively lifting the ball overhead to ensure the further accumulation of lean muscle mass. It is important to make the distinction that you are training to change your physical composition, and any improvement in actual performance is merely a by-product of the physical change you will have undergone. That is, if you have more stamina or can throw a ball faster and farther as a result of your training, it's a bonus but not the goal.

When I competed in bodybuilding, one area I would best many of my competitors was when we were turned to our sides. I couldn't wait for the judges to call "quarter turn to the right," because generally my competitors looked good from the front and the back but would literally thin out or disappear from the side. I beat them on thickness because I always believed in training for what I call a 3-D look. This look is

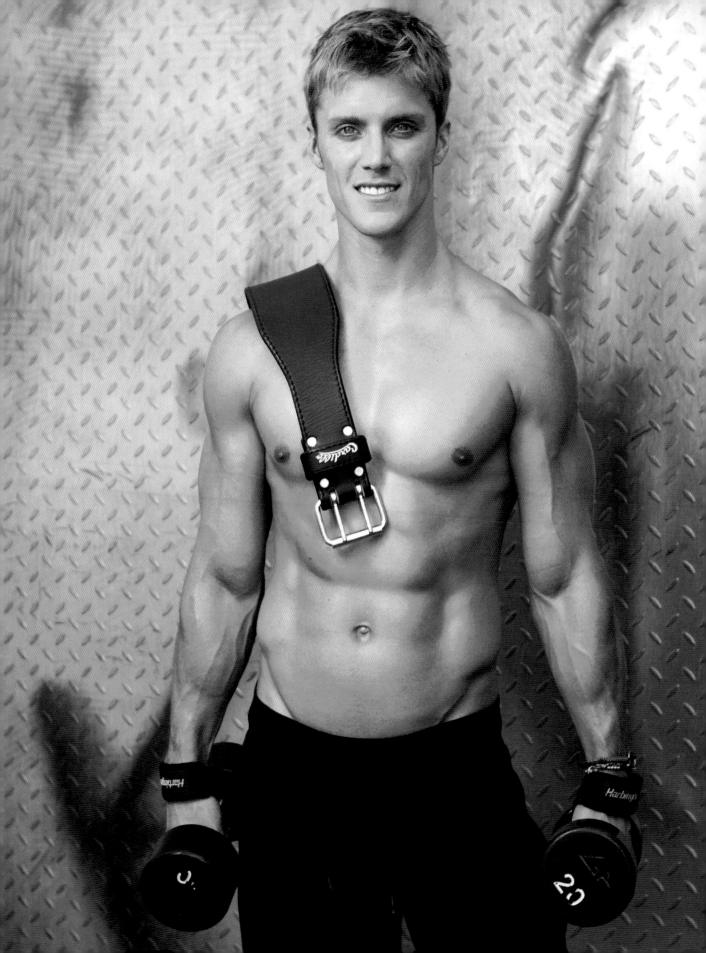

accomplished through the basics and foundational training: deadlifts, rows, squats and presses. The ectomorph may not have been born with genetically wide shoulders and may not have the wingspan of a 747, but he can indeed capture the eye with a pronounced thickness from the side.

You would be hard-pressed to build this 3-D look from machines alone. It's free weights that build mass. Machines certainly have their place in the ectomorph's workout, but they are limited by their preselected pathway of motion, which is much more isolating than free weights. Free weights, on the other hand, have no pre-selected pathway and require the addition of ancillary muscles for both support and execution during lifting. Compare athletes who regularly perform multi-joint exercises with free weights with those with machine-built bodies, and you will see a huge difference in terms of muscle fullness, thickness, and even hardness.

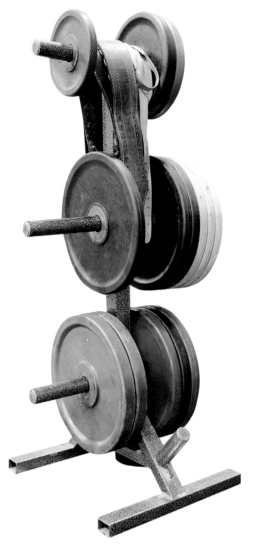

ANATOMY OF A REP

The repetition, or single performance of an exercise from start to finish, is simple yet vital to changing your body. The repetition consists of three parts: the negative, the positive, and the static. In the cause for renewed muscle growth, although all three are important, it is during the negative, or lowering of the weight (the descent during a bench press), that the majority of muscle breakdown occurs. This is why it is so important to always be in control of your repetitions—especially when lowering the weight and stretching muscles. It is very easy to go from muscle fatigue and failure to a muscle tear, so be cautious when selecting a weight, for you need to be able to complete the repetition. Growth will not occur with heavy negatives alone.

The positive, or lifting of the weight (ascension during a bench press), forces the muscle to action through a completed range of motion. Its execution should be explosive, in sharp contrast to the negative, though always controlled. Think of the negative as the cocking of the hammer on a gun and the positive as the firing of the bullet. Although the positive is not the strongest portion of the rep, its role is vital for muscular growth.

The static portion of an exercise is the fully contracted position of the repetition (the flexed position of a curl). This can be achieved in most exercises, most notably excluding the squat and deadlift. The static portion is perhaps the most abused and neglected part of a repetition. It is often skipped in an effort to finish a given set, or simply impossible when the given weight is too heavy, but it is important to achieve a peak contraction to not only fully engage and exhaust the muscles, but also to achieve optimal control and develop new muscle tissue.

TAKE MY BREATH AWAY

It is often discussed during vocal training, yoga, and most certainly childbirth, but during weight training the subject of breathing often only comes up somewhere between "How much do you bench?" and "How many times should I eat each day?" And breathing remains, in the scheme of things, a less glamorous subject than many others.

As for breathing during exercise, the first point is to simply continue doing so. You may find yourself holding your breath as you work out, and you may even think it will help with performance, but this is bad practice—and in extreme cases can actually lead to a heart attack.

Breathing comes down to two very simple things. First, you inhale on the negative (descent during a squat, for instance). Second, you exhale on the positive or execution of the repetition (ascent during a squat). The key is to utilize the breath as an offensive tactic. For example, when performing a heavy set of barbell rows, you will inhale slowly and deeply on the lowering of the bar and stretching of the lats, and then you will exhale forcefully as you pull the bar into your waist while thrusting your elbows forcefully behind you. The exhale helps to accentuate performance during both the positive and static portions of the repetition.

CHEATING

Although definitely a no-no when it comes to test-taking and relationships, in weight training or bodybuilding, cheating does have a place when applied appropriately. For our purposes, you will record achieving a target set only if you perform it honestly. But as you progress, besting those records becomes harder and less frequent. This is called the law of diminishing returns. And though lifting a new stimulus so that your muscles can adapt by growing is important, tension on the muscle is equally as important. After all, what good is a bench press that uses a surplus of an arched back and anterior shoulders to hoist up the load? The actual number of reps or sets may go up, but so too will your chance of injury, while your lean muscle mass will not increase.

And yet as a set progresses and the muscle at hand gets ever-closer to imminent temporary muscular failure, the tendency is to kick in with nearby ancillary muscle groups to garner a few extra reps. And while you might not record those reps as legitimate in your training diary, this temporary assistance will allow you to travel where you have not previously, and that is progress. The next time you are faced with the same load, chances are high that you will cleanly perform those new reps.

Let's say you're performing a set of barbell curls strictly by keeping your elbows in, employing a full range of motion (especially on the negative), and maintaining relatively good posture. As it becomes increasingly more difficult and soon nearly impossible to complete a full repetition and close the arms to full flexion, now is the time to add just enough assistance from the lower back to complete, not take over, the repetition. The key to cheating is to employ it only near the end of a set when possible muscular failure has been achieved, and even then offer only enough assistance from ancillary muscle groups to get the job done, not complete it on its own.

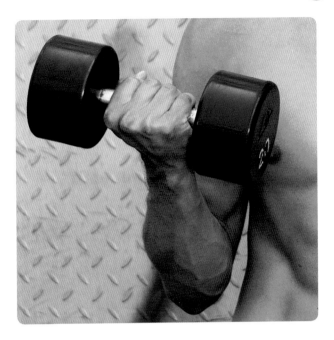

REST

Rest and recuperation are as vital to your success as their cousins, nutrition and training. A muscle can be worked and fed, yet without sufficient rest to repair and grow it may actually revert backward and risk possible injury. Off days have been placed within your workout program to allow for ample recovery from the stresses that weight training places upon you. It does little good to train legs one day and to go out dancing the next if new muscle mass is your primary goal.

THE TOOLS

In powerlifting, the single focus is to move a given weight from A to B to receive a green light from the judges. But in your endeavor here, bodybuilding, the goal is to place as much tension upon a working muscle through a full range of motion. The actual amount of weight used is merely a tool, not the end result, so there are certain aids that you can employ to help maximize not only the loads handled but to also keep the tension on a given muscle for longer periods of time through repetitions. This creates more temporary muscle fatigue and, ultimately, growth.

For the sake of pure muscle building, utilize what I call The Big 3: belts, straps, and chalk. These three training peripherals will in some instances, protect, fortify, reinforce, and allow you to go beyond failure or the norm of what is commonly referred to as "raw." Going raw is usually a term reserved for powerlifting meets in which outside elements are not used. Here you have no limits or restrictions.

BELTS

My personal favorite. For me the weight-lifting belt is mandatory on any type of bent-over row, bent-over lateral, overhead press, heavy curl, or squatting movement. The snug support braced against the back ensures optimal confidence and performance.

STRAPS

The greatest plus about lifting straps that wrap around the wrists—besides their portability—is that they ensure that the muscles give out before your grip does. This equates to a firmer and more solid grip on the bar, extra reps and, ultimately, more muscle growth.

CHALK

Chalk can be a real asset in helping you lift. Look at the size of your hands and forearms. Now look at your back. Obviously your back is much larger, yet your hands and forearms are links to your back, and they must be able to hold on to a weight. You need all the support and fortification you can get for those heavy poundages and extra growth-inducing reps. On a set of deadlifts, chalk locks in a grip so tight that you may have to be pried from the bar at the conclusion of your set. Still, chalk is definitely messy and a no-no in many gyms.

FOAM ROLLING

Foam rolling has become a standard modality of exercise today, as commonplace as sipping a protein shake post workout, and for good reason: foam rolling, or myofascial release therapy as it is technically called, breaks up restricted muscles, improves performance and flexibility, and encourages recovery at a fraction of the cost of a massage therapist. It can also be used nearly anywhere. Muscles with compromised function are called "knots" or "trigger points" and can be rolled out manually through self-treatment. Foam rolling also serves as an excellent precursor to actual exercise.

Although the tendency is to tighten muscles when pressure is applied

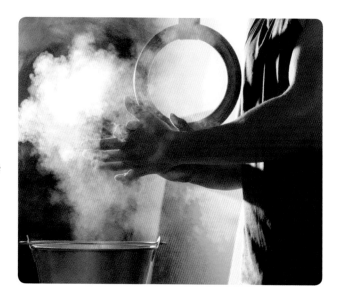

to an already restricted state, it is important to try to relax as you are rolling. Pausing at unusually tight areas while you glide back and forth gently will cause muscles to loosen and the pain to be released. Here, time or repetitions are not important. Focus on releasing the fascia, a thin tissue that covers muscles that can become shortened and restricted, which can cause an imbalance and uneven tightness in surrounding tissues.

Myofascial release, often slightly discomforting to mildly painful at first, essentially resets order and balance to the body and helps muscles properly fire and perform, pain-free. With regular practice, you'll quickly adapt to rolling and begin to enjoy its myriad benefits. The ectomorph program calls for foam rolling to take place prior to your workout session.

STRETCHING

We all know that stretching is indeed beneficial, but we may not know why or even when it is best to stretch. Stretching helps to promote a fuller range of motion in muscle tissue, reduce muscle tension, increase energy levels, and increase blood circulation to name a few of its many benefits. Stretching is so important that we do it without even thinking. Upon waking up, we instinctively stretch our bodies to prepare them for motion and elongate that which has been in a state of flexion for some hours. Animals naturally stretch upon waking as they too prepare for motion.

Stretching prior to exercise was long considered the best time to stretch. Although some light stretching prior to working out is okay, the problem here is that muscles at this time are not warmed up—they are cold and nonpliable. Stretch or pull on them

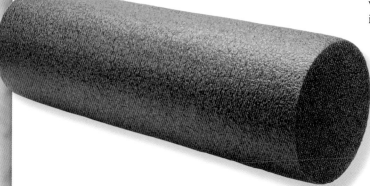

too firmly, and you risk a tear. Indeed, the best time to stretch is both during and after your training when your muscles are warm, looser, and more pliable.

Consider this: the more flexible you are, the greater your range of motion in a given exercise and the more muscle tissue you can develop. The ectomorph program calls for stretching to take place following your workout session.

CARDIO

For your goals and the purposes and scope of this book, the subject of cardiovascular exercise is almost a nonissue. The main goal of cardio as it pertains to the realm of aesthetic fitness is not about improved performance nor is it about burning calories, which is the common belief, but rather to help speed up the metabolism and utilize stored adipose (fat) as fuel. Speeding up the metabolism is not something an ectomorph usually needs. Your main goal is putting on quality body weight, namely muscle tissue, so cardio is far down on the list of important initiatives.

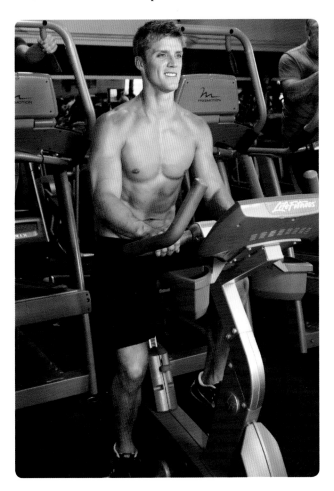

The term *cardiovascular* pertains to any activity 20 minutes or longer in duration that involves the heart. Weight training is very stop and go, so it falls under a different branch of exercise. What many people fail to realize, however, is that weight training tends to burn more calories than a typical cardio session and will certainly do far more in terms of hardening the body or enhancing one's shape than cardio alone will. Because a strong heart and an efficient metabolism are important, some semblance of cardio has been added to your program. It must be undertaken at the end of your weight training routine—never before it, as this will deplete your glycogen or stored carbohydrates that would normally be used for weight training. You'd be left with little gas in the tank for the all-important weight-training portion of your program.

Where people run into trouble is performing cardio too strenuously and too often in an effort to lean up but what actually happens is this intense performance of cardio often results in a ravenous state whereby the subject winds up eating more food than normal, specifically high-glycemic carbs, and winds up gaining more weight. This is why you see so many heavy or overweight cardio enthusiasts.

In summation, for your purposes here, a few sessions of cardio are placed within your training regimen a few times per week, for no longer than 20 minutes, and at a low intensity for some semblance of cardiovascular efficacy. By low intense, pretend someone is next to you while performing your cardio. If you can't comfortably exchange dialogue with them, the cardio is too intense and could be cutting into your recuperation and ultimately affect your muscle gains. I would suggest avoiding running, intense stair climbing, or VersaClimbing; in short, any over-intensified cardio session. I find that the ectomorph responds favorably to the stationary bike, Precor elliptical machine, or treadmill on a sight incline for a walk.

In short—Cardio: go through the motions. Weight training: give your all. Nutrition: eat consistently to gain. Recuperation: rest, repair, grow, and build.

PHOTOGRAPHS

Take them. From all four sides of your body on the very first day that you begin this program. And don't cheat by "pumping up" first. Take them cold. It doesn't matter if you don't have a tan, or are too hairy or want a "better starting point." Take them now and then put them away. They are for your eyes only. Do it, no matter how painful it may seem. Shirt off too. Shorts and socks only.

THE WORKOUTS

This is the chapter you've probably flipped to first, and for good reason: it's the map that leads to the treasure that is the new you. Your workouts are covered in their entirety—workouts that will take you from skinny to beefy in three progressive phases.

HOW IT WORKS

Each four-week phase covers the major muscle groups of the body, training each group once per week. What largely differs between the phases are extra exercises or substitute exercises as you advance and are able to handle heavier poundages and more progressive lifts.

Of particular importance is that you are firing from the targeted muscles. If you can perform an impressive bench press but feel the majority of firing power from the shoulders and triceps as opposed to the pectorals, your effort is wasted and does little in terms of aesthetics. Also, there must exist a natural progression in weights handled. If you are still using the same

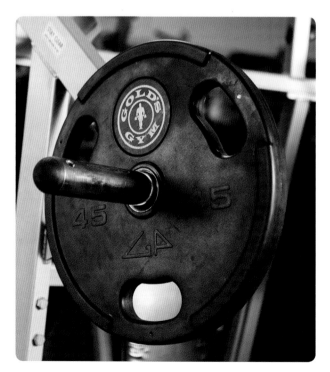

poundages in week 12 as you were in week 1, little to no muscle growth has occurred, no matter how "different" the training regimen may be. And although some people may "confuse" their muscles by changing workouts and even goals, this does nothing to add lean muscle mass to your frame.

What follows below are the three phases of workouts listed in detail. Be sure to complete each phase for the prescribed 4-week period before proceeding to the next. As you progress, you will gain muscle control, an understanding of the proper muscle-building angles, and a mind-to-muscle connection. That is, you will feel the correct muscles firing from the first repetition—and that only comes with experience. Once completing the 12-week program, aside from having made noticeable improvements in both muscle size and strength, one look in the mirror will most assuredly be cause for you to continue your journey.

WORKOUT SMART

The focus on abdominals has been included to offer a more well-rounded and complete training program, but it is important to note that these muscles are used in just about every lift, and so a surplus amount of direct abdominal work is unnecessary to develop them.

Again, only trace amounts of cardiovascular exercise are listed because the ectomorph is primarily concerned with putting weight on, not taking it off. Performing cardio is largely recommended so that you gain a semblance of cardiovascular conditioning and process nutrients more efficiently.

The foam-rolling exercises are placed to precede your actual weight training. These will warm up tight and restricted muscles. The stretches provided are recommended for after your weight training, when your muscles are warm and pliable.

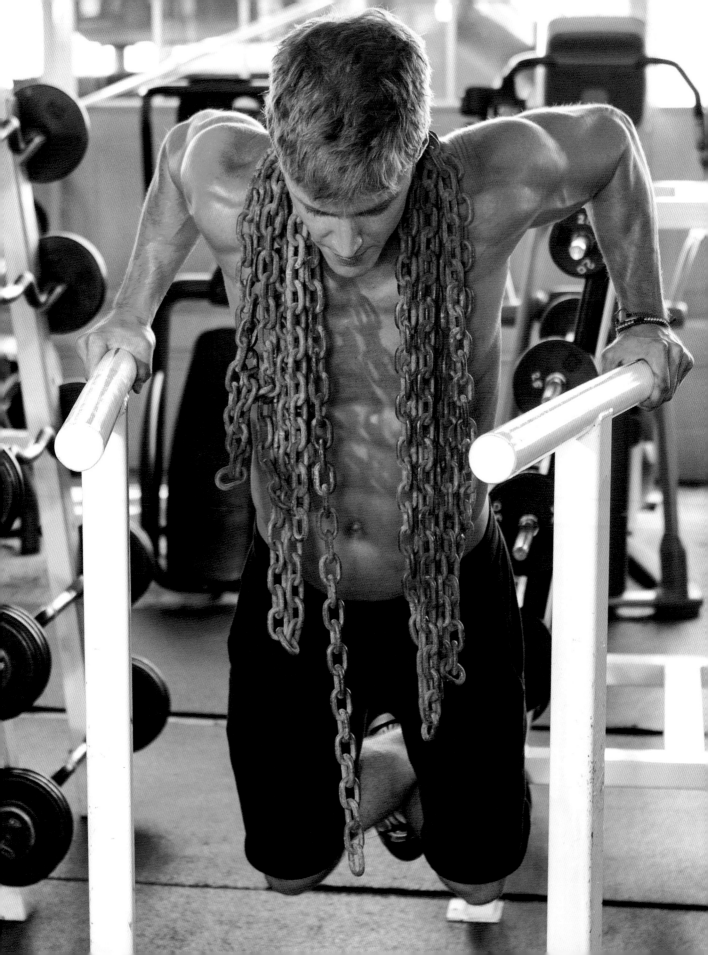

PHASE 1
WEEKS 1–4

MONDAY
Chest/Back/Abdominals + 20-minute cardio

Foam Roller Exercises:
- Lower Back
- Upper Back
- Latissimus

Exercises:
- Incline Dumbbell Press *superset* with
  Sumo Deadlift 3 x 6–10
- Flat Barbell Press *superset* with Barbell Row
  3 x 6–10
- Hammer Strength Incline Press *superset*
  with Single-Arm Machine Row 2 x 8–10
- Flat Dumbbell Fly *superset* with
  Reverse-Grip Pulldown 2 x 8–10
- Seated Leg Tuck *superset* with
  Twisting Crunch 2 x 25

Stretches:
- Kneeling Lat Stretch
- Lower Back Stretch
- Chest Stretch

TUESDAY
REST

WEDNESDAY
Legs

Foam Roller Exercises:
- Quadriceps
- Adductors
- IT Band
- Glutes/Piriformis
- Hamstrings
- Calves

Exercises:
- Barbell Squat 3 x 10–12
- Leg Press 3 x 10–12
- Smith Machine Split Squat 2 x 10–12 per leg
- Lying Leg Curl 3 x 10–12
- Stiff-Legged Deadlift 3 x 10–12
- Seated Calf Raise 3 x 12–15

Stretches:
- Shin Stretch
- Toe Touch
- Calf Stretch

THURSDAY
REST

FRIDAY
**Shoulders/Arms/Abdominals
+ 20-minute cardio**

Foam Roller Exercises:
- Upper Back
- Latissimus

Exercises:
- Hammer Strength Shoulder Press 3 x 6–10
- Dumbbell Shrug 3 x 6–10
- Seated Lateral Raise 3 x 8–10
- Bent-Over Lateral Raise 3 x 8–10
- EZ-Curl Barbell Curl *superset* with
  Vertical Dip 2 x 8–10
- Alternate Hammer Curl *superset* with Dumbbell
  Skull Crusher 2 x 8–10
- Incline Dumbbell Curl *superset* with Bar
  Pushdown 2 x 10–12
- Seated Leg Tuck *superset* with
  Twisting Crunch 2 x 25

Stretches:
- Shoulder Stretch
- Biceps Stretch
- Triceps Stretch

SATURDAY
REST

SUNDAY
REST

FOLLOWING THE EXERCISE INSTRUCTIONS
Each exercise lists the number of sets and
reps. An example reads: "Dumbbell Shrug
3 x 6–10." This means "perform three sets of
6 to 10 repetitions." When you see *superset*, that
means to perform two or more exercises back
to back without pausing. An example would
include "Incline Dumbbell Press *superset* with Bar
Pushdown 2 x 10–12." This translates to "perform
two sets of both exercises back to back for 10 to
12 repetitions per set."

PHASE 2
WEEKS 5–8

MONDAY
Back/Abdominals + 20-minute cardio

Foam Roller Exercises:
- Lower Back
- Upper Back
- Latissimus

Exercises:
- Sumo Deadlift 3 x 6–10 or Deadlift 3 x 6–10
- Barbell Row 3 x 6–10 or T-Bar Row 3 x 6–10
- Single-Arm Machine Row 3 x 8–10
- Machine Pullover 3 x 8–10
- Reverse-Grip Pulldown 3 x 8–10
- Seated Leg Tuck *superset* with
     Twisting Crunch 2 x 25

Stretches:
- Kneeling Lat Stretch
- Lower Back Stretch

TUESDAY
Chest/Biceps

Exercises:
- Incline Dumbbell Press 3 x 6–10
- Flat Barbell Press 3 x 6–10
- Hammer Strength Incline Press 3 x 8–10
- Flat Dumbbell Fly 2 x 8–10
- Cable Crossover 2 x 10–12
- EZ-Curl Barbell Curl 2 x 8–10
- Preacher Curl 2 x 10–12
- Incline Dumbbell Curl 2 x 10–12

Stretches:
- Chest Stretch
- Biceps Stretch

WEDNESDAY
REST

THURSDAY
Legs

Foam Roller Exercises:
- Quadriceps
- Adductors
- IT Band
- Glutes/Piriformis
- Hamstrings
- Calves

Exercises:
- Barbell Squat 3 x 10–12
- Leg Press 3 x 10–12
- Smith Machine Split Squat 2 x 10–12 per leg
- Leg Extension 2 x 10–12
- Lying Leg Curl 3 x 10–12
- Seated Leg Curl 2 x 10–12
- Stiff-Legged Deadlift 2 x 10–12
     or Kettlebell Stiff-Legged Deadlift 2 x 10–12
- Seated Calf Raise 3 x 12–15

Stretches:
- Shin Stretch
- Toe Touch
- Calf Stretch

FRIDAY
Shoulders/Triceps/Abdominals
+ 20-minute cardio

Foam Roller Exercises:
- Upper Back
- Latissimus

Exercises:
- Hammer Strength Shoulder Press 3 x 6–10
- Barbell Power Clean 2 x 6–8
     or Kettlebell One-Arm Clean 2 x 6–8
- Dumbbell Shrug 3 x 6–10
- Seated Lateral Raise 3 x 8–10
- Bent-Over Lateral Raise 3 x 8–10
- Vertical Dip 2 x 8–10
- Dumbbell Skull Crusher 2 x 8–10
- Bar Pushdown 2 x 10–12
- Machine Triceps Extension 2 x 10–12
- Seated Leg Tuck *superset* with
     Twisting Crunch 2 x 25

Stretches:
- Shoulder Stretch
- Triceps Stretch

SATURDAY
REST

SUNDAY
REST

PHASE 3
WEEKS 9–12

MONDAY
Back/Abdominals + 20-minute cardio

Foam Roller Exercises:
• Lower Back
• Upper Back
• Latissimus

Exercises:
• Deadlift 3 x 6–10
• Hyperextension 2 x 12–15
• T-Bar Row 3 x 6–10
• Kettlebell One-Arm Row or
    Single-Arm Low Row 2 x 8–10
• Machine Pullover 3 x 8–10
• Reverse-Grip Pulldown 2 x 8–10
• Pull-Up 2 x 8–10
• Seated Leg Tuck *superset* with
    Twisting Crunch 2 x 25

Stretches:
• Kneeling Lat Stretch
• Lower Back Stretch

TUESDAY
Chest/Biceps/Abdominals

Exercises:
• Incline Dumbbell Press 3 x 6–10
• Flat Barbell Press 3 x 6–10
• Hammer Strength Incline Press 3 x 8–10
• Flat Dumbbell Fly 2 x 8–10
• Cable Crossover 2 x 10–12
• EZ-Curl Barbell Curl 2 x 8–10
• Alternate Hammer Curl 2x 8–10
• Preacher Curl 2 x 10–12
• Incline Dumbbell Curl 2 x 10–12
• Seated Leg Tuck *superset* with
    Twisting Crunch 2 x 25

Stretches:
• Chest Stretch
• Biceps Stretch

WEDNESDAY
REST

THURSDAY
Legs + 20-minute cardio

Foam Roller Exercises:
• Quadriceps
• Adductors
• IT Band
• Glutes/Piriformis
• Hamstrings
• Calves

Exercises:
• Barbell Squat 3 x 10–12
• Reverse Hack Squat 2 x 10–12
• Leg Press 3 x 10–12
• Smith Machine Split Squat 2 x 10–12 per leg
• Leg Extension 2 x 10–12
• Lying Leg Curl 3 x 10–12
• Seated Leg Curl 2 x 10–12
• Kettlebell Stiff-Legged Deadlift 2 x 10–12
• Seated Calf Raises 3 x 12–15
• Tibia Raise 2 x 12–15

Stretches:
• Shin Stretch
• Toe Touch
• Calf Stretch

FRIDAY
Shoulders/Triceps/Abdominals + 20-minute cardio

Foam Roller Exercises:
• Upper Back
• Latissimus

Exercises:
• Hammer Strength Shoulder Press
    or Standing Military Press 3 x 6–10
• Kettlebell One-Arm Clean and Press 2 x 6–8
• Dumbbell Shrug 3 x 6–10
• Seated Lateral Raise 3 x 8–10
• Standing Single-Arm Lateral Raise 2 x 10–12
• Bent-Over Lateral Raise 3 x 8–10
• Vertical Dip 2 x 8–10
• Dumbbell Skull Crusher 2 x 8–10
• Bar Pushdown 2 x 10–12
• Overhead Rope Extension 2 x 10–12
• Machine Triceps Extension 2 x 10–12
• Seated Leg Tuck *superset* with
    Twisting Crunch 2 x 25

Stretches:
• Shoulder Stretch
• Triceps Stretch

SATURDAY
REST

SUNDAY
REST

UPPER BACK

PROGRESSION

1 Begin in a reclined position with a foam roller beneath your upper back. Fold your hands across your chest, and bend your legs.

2 With your head and neck in a neutral position and your abdominal muscles stabilized, gently roll up and down from just below your trapezius muscles to the top of your rhomboids, being sure to avoid rolling over your neck. Roll for 30 to 60 seconds.

MUSCLE ACTION
Primary activation
- trapezius
- rhomboids

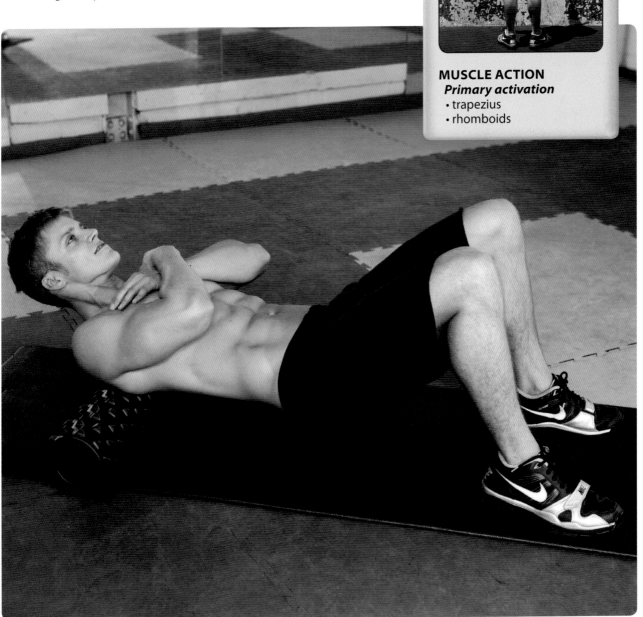

LOWER BACK

PROGRESSION

1 Begin in a reclined position with a foam roller placed beneath your middle back. Place your hands behind your head, and bend your knees.

2 With your head and neck in a neutral position and your abdominal muscles stabilized, gently roll up and down from just above your hips to just below your ribs, being sure to avoid rolling over your lower spine. Roll for 30 to 60 seconds.

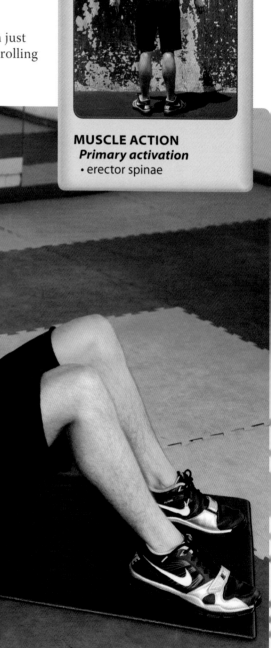

MUSCLE ACTION
Primary activation
• erector spinae

LATISSIMUS

PROGRESSION

1 Begin on your side with the roller placed just beneath your armpit against the latissimus dorsi muscle. Bend your top leg, planting your foot on the floor behind the knee of your bottom leg. Keep your bottom leg straight.

2 Position your front arm straight over the top of the roller. Place the opposite hand on the ground in front of you for support.

3 Gently rock forward and backward. Roll for 30 to 60 seconds, and then repeat on the opposite side.

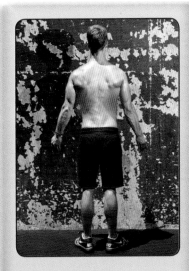

MUSCLE ACTION
Primary activation
• latissimus dorsi

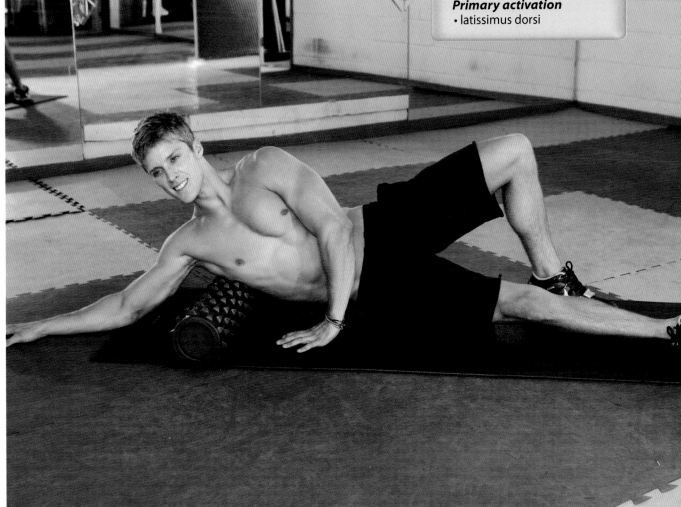

QUADRICEPS

PROGRESSION

1 Begin facedown with the roller placed underneath your thighs, your legs straight, and your torso braced in the plank position supported on your forearms.

2 Roll from just above your knees to just below your hips, allowing your toes to drag. Roll for 30 to 60 seconds.

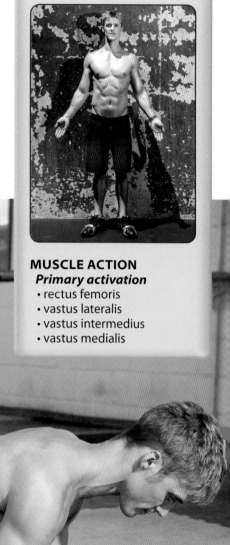

MUSCLE ACTION
Primary activation
• rectus femoris
• vastus lateralis
• vastus intermedius
• vastus medialis

ADDUCTORS
PROGRESSION

1 Begin facedown with your torso braced in the plank position with the roller placed vertically beneath you and with one knee resting on the floor and the opposite groin pressed against the roller.

2 Slowly move your hips side to side as you roll along the length of the adductor muscles. Roll for 30 to 60 seconds, and then repeat on the opposite side.

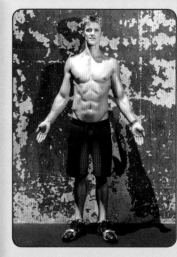

MUSCLE ACTION
Primary activation
• hip adductors

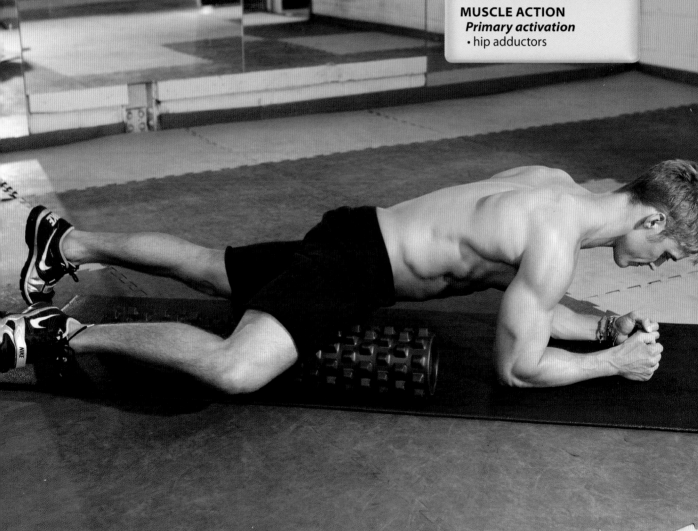

IT BAND

PROGRESSION

1 Begin on your side with the roller placed beneath you between your knee and your hip and with your arms propped to support your torso. Keep your lower leg extended with the foot braced against the floor, and cross your top leg over it so that your foot is planted flat on the ground.

2 With the assistance of your legs and arms, roll the length of your IT band along the upper portion of your thigh to just above your knee. Roll for 30 to 60 seconds, and then repeat on the opposite side.

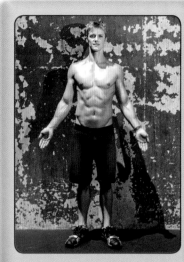

MUSCLE ACTION
Primary activation
• iliotibial band

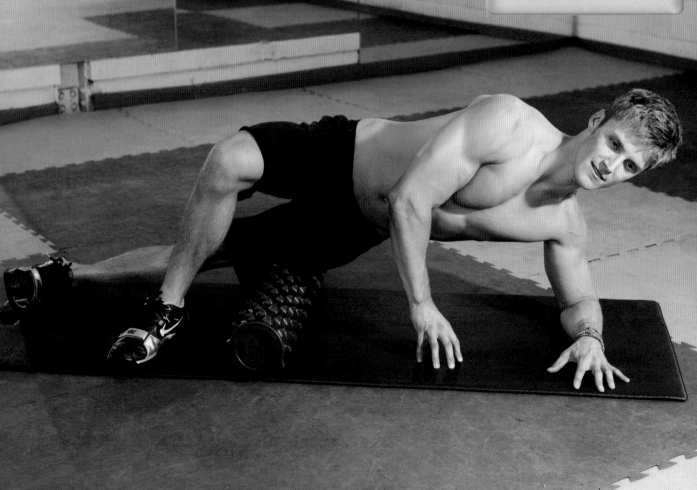

GLUTES/PIRIFORMIS

PROGRESSION

1 Begin seated with the roller placed beneath your glutes and your arms behind you for support.

2 Cross one ankle over the opposite thigh, shifting your weight to that same side.

3 Roll forward and backward over the muscle for 30 to 60 seconds, and then repeat on the opposite side.

MUSCLE ACTION
Primary activation
- gluteus maximus
- piriformis

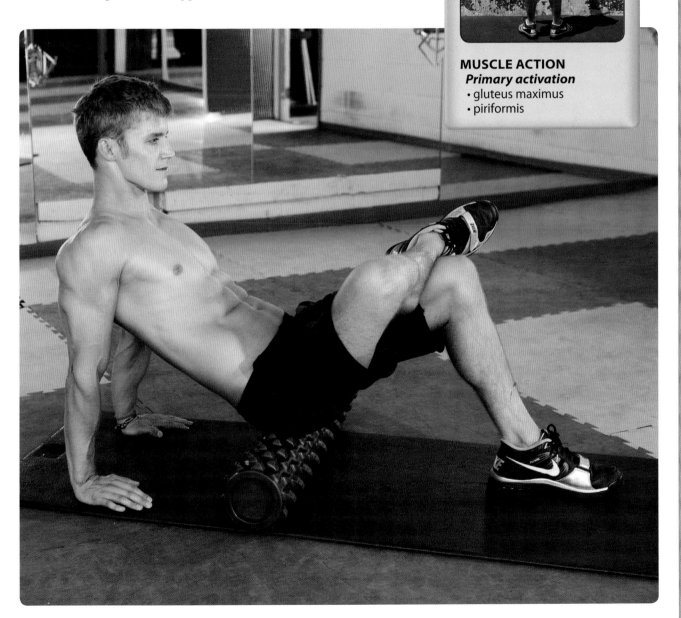

HAMSTRINGS

PROGRESSION

1 Begin seated with the roller placed beneath your upper hamstring muscles below your glutes. Prop your arms behind you for support.

2 Start by rolling from just above the knees to just below your pelvis. Roll for 30 to 60 seconds.

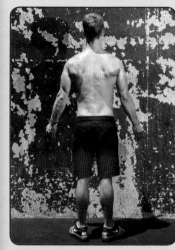

MUSCLE ACTION
Primary activation
- biceps femoris
- semitendinosus
- semimembranosus

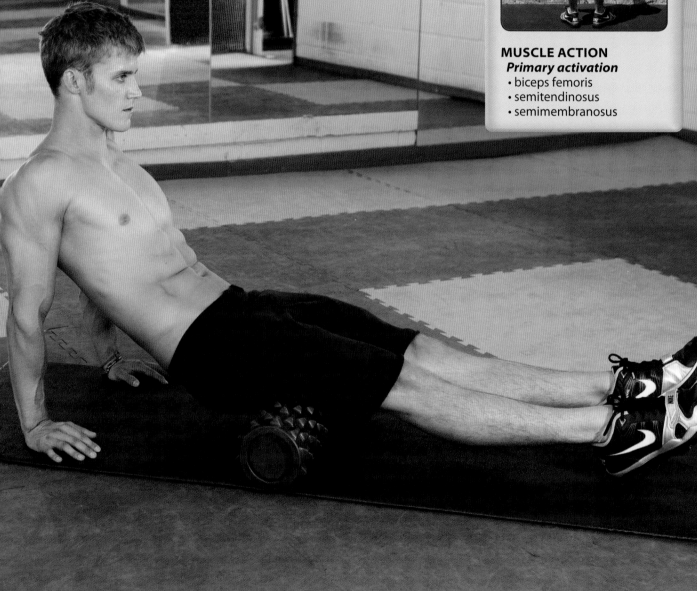

CALVES
PROGRESSION

1 Begin in a seated position with the roller placed beneath your calves and your arms propped behind you for support.

2 Start by rolling over your calf muscles from just below your knees to just above your ankles. Roll for 30 to 60 seconds.

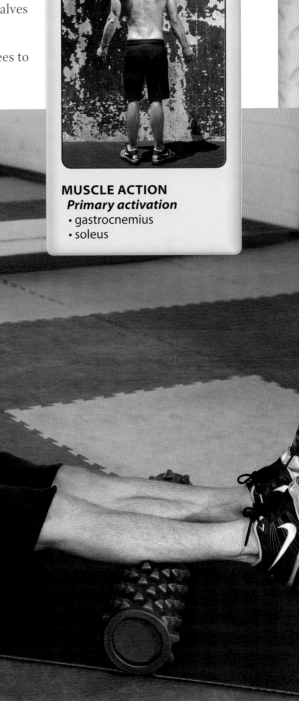

MUSCLE ACTION
Primary activation
• gastrocnemius
• soleus

SUMO DEADLIFT

PROGRESSION

1 Begin standing in front of a weighted barbell with your feet very wide apart and your toes facing slightly outward.

2 Squat down and grab the barbell with an overhand grip, your wrists in line with your elbows. Your chest should be directly above the bar, your spine straight and your head up.

3 Push through your heels as you stand erect with the barbell held below you at arm's length, and then lower carefully to the ground for 6 to 10 repetitions.

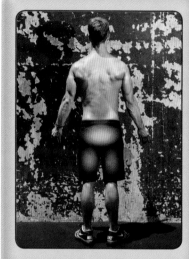

MUSCLE ACTION
Primary activation
- erector spinae
- hamstrings
- gluteus maximus
- rectus abdominis
- quadriceps

Ancillary activation
- trapezius
- biceps
- wrist and forearm flexors
- wrist and forearm extensors

PROPER FORM
Do
- Maintain a flat back throughout the movement.
- Keep the weight bar close to your body.
- Stand completely erect at the top of the movement.

Avoid
- Rounding your back.
- Slamming down the weight.
- Pushing through the toes.

MODIFICATIONS
Beginner
- Use the weight bar only.

Advanced
- Take a closer stance to increase range of motion.

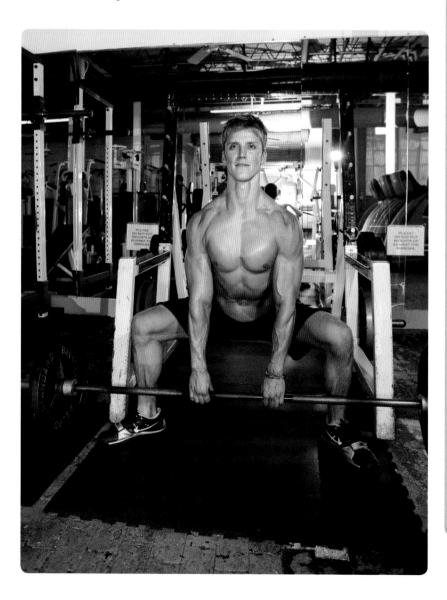

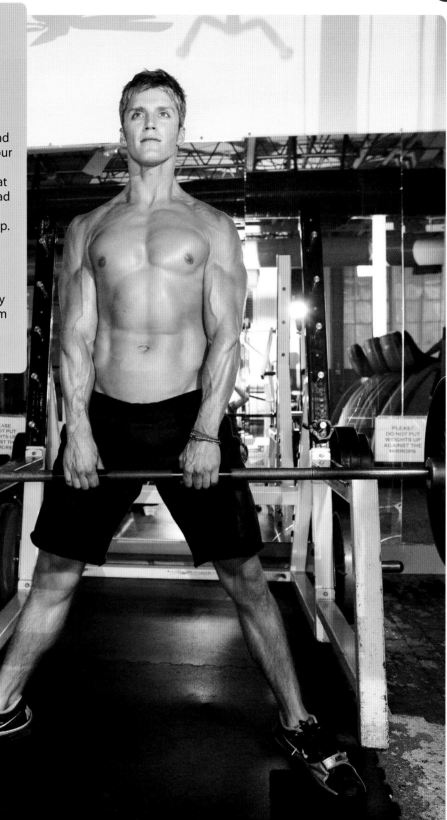

BACK TIPS

A strong back is crucial, and it takes a complex group of muscles working together to support your spine. These important muscles, including the erector spinae group and the large latissimus dorsi, help you to hold yourself upright and allow you to twist and bend your trunk. When training the back, think of the hands as hooks that are latching onto the bar instead of squeezing too firmly, which will weaken and dilute your grip. Whether the motion is pulling down or rowing backward, move your arms as if you were elbowing an invisible person behind you in order to properly contract the lats. Never perform a behind-the-neck pulldown because this can put undue strain on the rotator muscles.

DEADLIFT

PROGRESSION

1 Begin standing in front of a weighted barbell with your feet shoulder-width apart. Hold the bar with an alternating grip with one hand overhand and one underhand.

2 Squat down with your chest directly above the bar, your spine straight and your head up.

3 Push through your heels as you stand erect with the barbell held below you at arm's length, and then lower carefully to the ground for 6 to 10 repetitions.

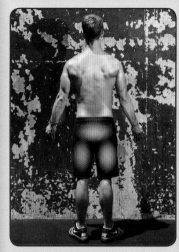

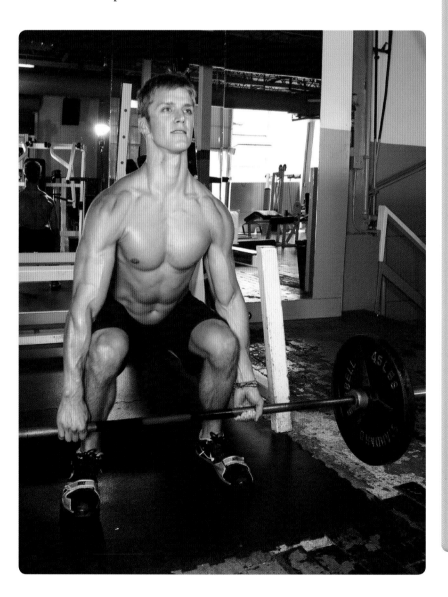

MUSCLE ACTION
Primary activation
- erector spinae
- hamstrings
- gluteus maximus
- rectus abdominis
- quadriceps

Ancillary activation
- trapezius
- biceps brachii
- wrist and forearm flexors
- wrist and forearm extensors

PROPER FORM
Do
- Maintain a flat back throughout the movement.
- Keep the weight bar close to your body.
- Stand completely erect at the top of the movement.

Avoid
- Rounding your back.
- Slamming down the weight.
- Pushing through the toes.

MODIFICATIONS
Beginner
- Use the weight bar only.

Advanced
- Take a closer stance to increase range of motion.

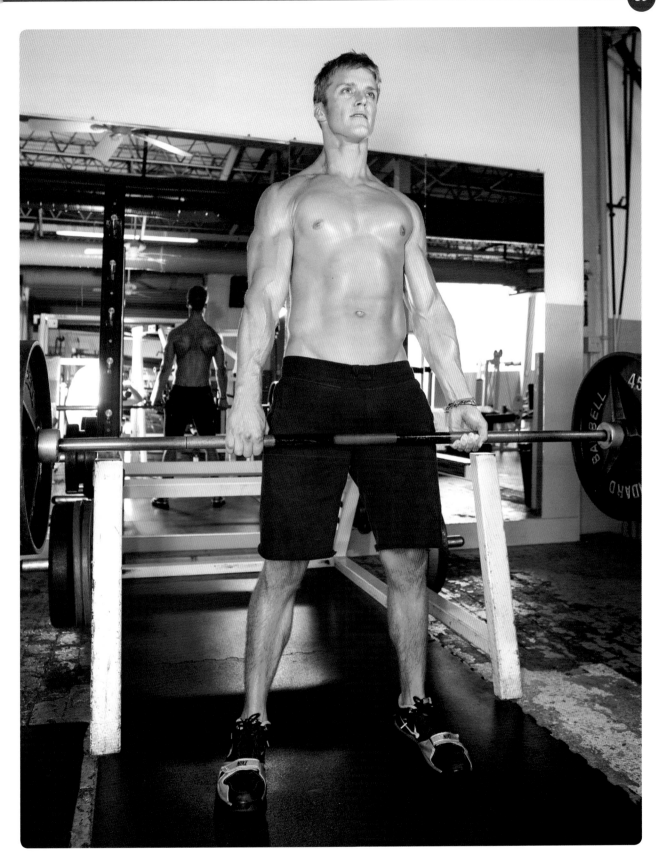

HYPEREXTENSION

PROGRESSION

1 Begin with your pelvis and thighs braced against the pad of a hyperextension machine. Press your heels against the leg support.

2 Fold your arms across your chest, and bend at the waist so that your face is parallel to the ground.

3 Raise your torso until your body is one straight line and parallel to the ground.

4 Lower your torso, and then repeat for 12 to 15 repetitions.

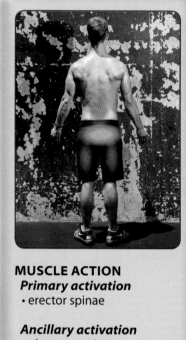

MUSCLE ACTION
Primary activation
• erector spinae

Ancillary activation
• gluteus maximus
• hamstrings

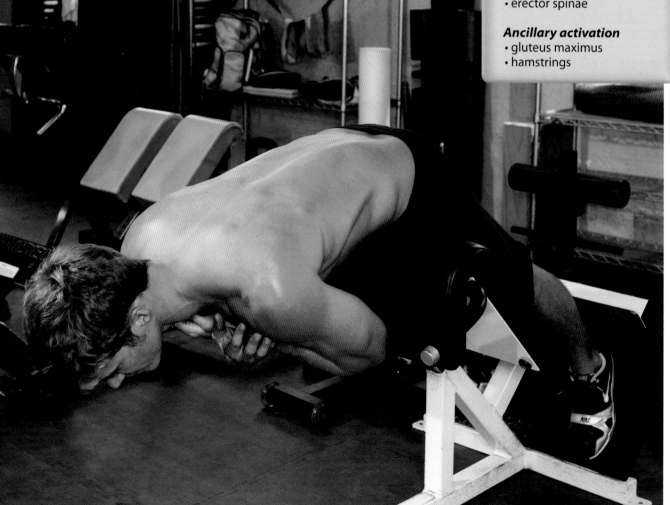

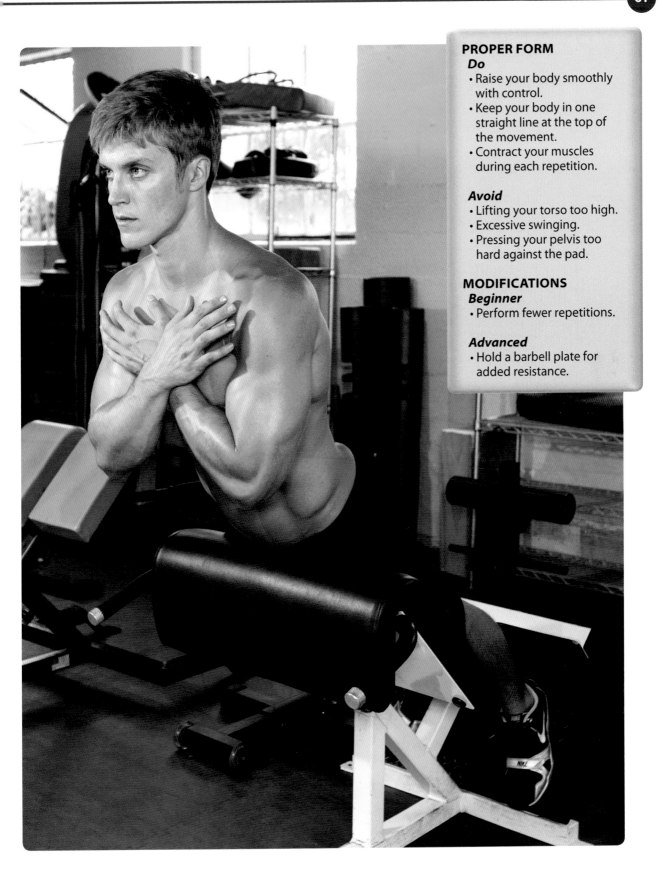

PROPER FORM

Do
- Raise your body smoothly with control.
- Keep your body in one straight line at the top of the movement.
- Contract your muscles during each repetition.

Avoid
- Lifting your torso too high.
- Excessive swinging.
- Pressing your pelvis too hard against the pad.

MODIFICATIONS

Beginner
- Perform fewer repetitions.

Advanced
- Hold a barbell plate for added resistance.

BARBELL ROW

PROGRESSION

1 Begin holding a barbell at arm's length with a overhand shoulder-width grip. Bend your knees slightly, and push out your rear as you lean forward at the waist until your back is slightly above parallel to the ground.

2 Pull your arms back as if you were rowing the bar into your midriff, tightly contracting your latissimus dorsi muscles.

3 Lower the barbell back down to full extension, and then repeat for 6 to 10 repetitions.

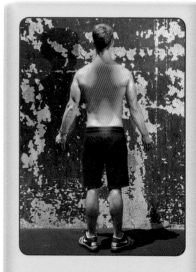

MUSCLE ACTION
Primary activation
- latissimus dorsi
- trapezius
- rhomboids

Ancillary activation
- biceps brachii
- rear deltoids
- erector spinae
- wrist and forearm flexors
- wrist and forearm extensors

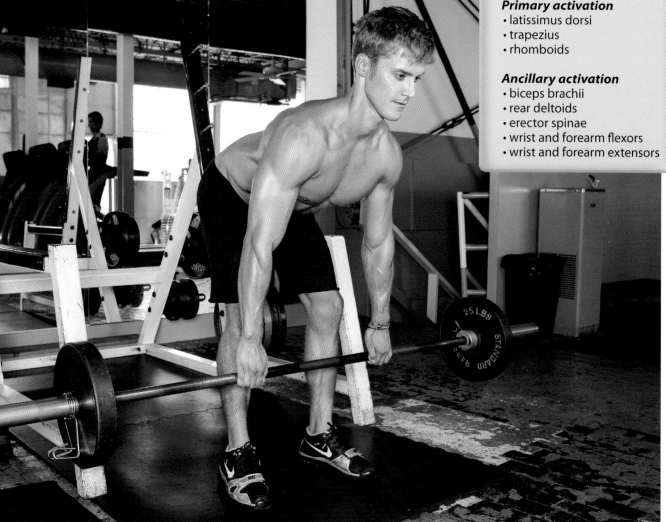

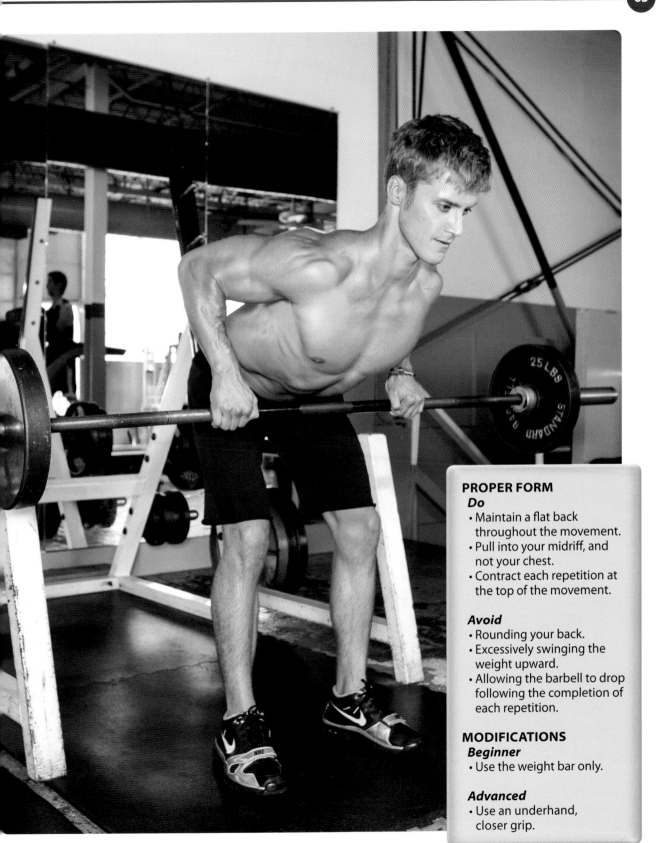

PROPER FORM
Do
- Maintain a flat back throughout the movement.
- Pull into your midriff, and not your chest.
- Contract each repetition at the top of the movement.

Avoid
- Rounding your back.
- Excessively swinging the weight upward.
- Allowing the barbell to drop following the completion of each repetition.

MODIFICATIONS
Beginner
- Use the weight bar only.

Advanced
- Use an underhand, closer grip.

T-BAR ROW

PROGRESSION

1 Stand before a makeshift T-bar row: a V-bar attachment hooked into the end of an Olympic bar with the other end anchored in a corner.

2 Take a neutral grip with your palms facing each other, and pull the bar inward to your abdomen.

3 Contract your latissimus dorsi and middle back muscles at the top of the movement, and then return to the starting position. Repeat for 6 to 10 repetitions.

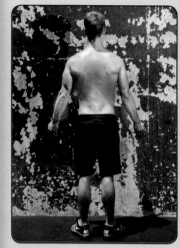

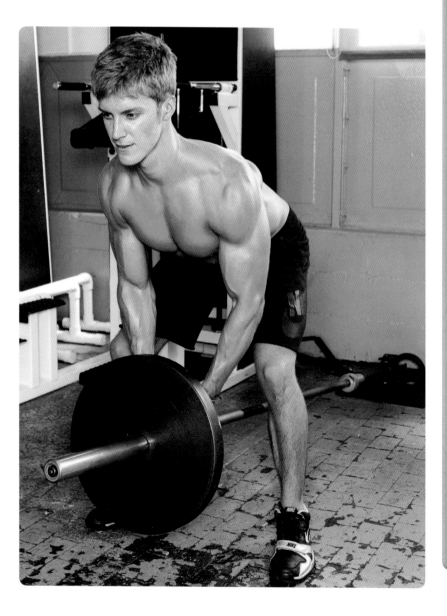

MUSCLE ACTION
Primary activation
- latissimus dorsi
- middle back

Ancillary activation
- biceps brachii
- rhomboids
- posterior deltoids
- wrist and forearm flexors
- wrist and forearm extensors

PROPER FORM
Do
- Maintain a flat back throughout the movement.
- Pull into your abdomen, and not your chest.
- Contract your muscles at the top of each repetition.

Avoid
- Rounding your back.
- Excessively swinging the weight.
- Allowing the weight to drop following the completion of each repetition.

MODIFICATIONS
Beginner
- Use a lighter weight.

Advanced
- Use one arm at a time.

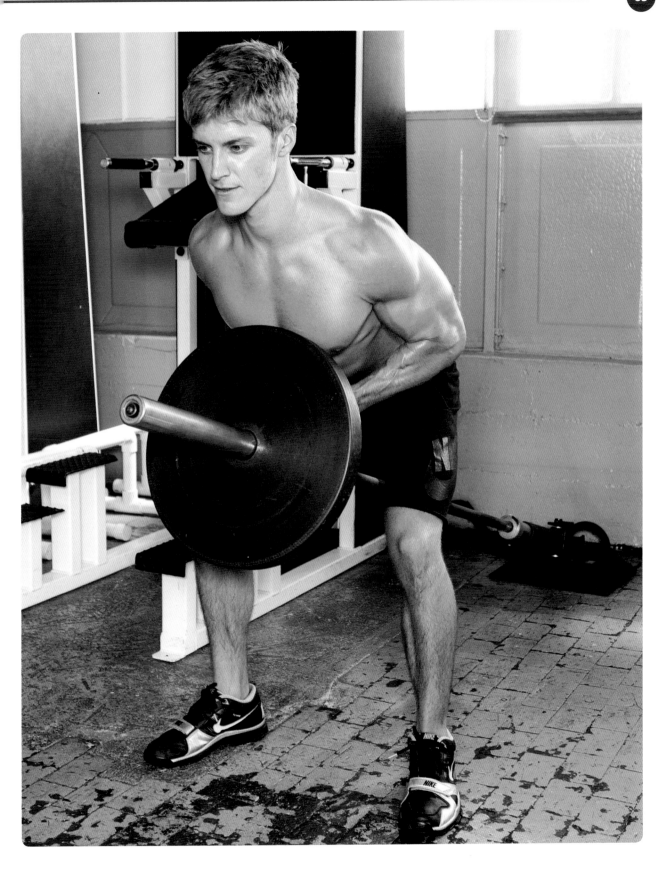

SINGLE-ARM MACHINE ROW

PROGRESSION

1 Begin in a seated position on a Hammer Strength row machine with the seat adjusted to a height at which your elbows will come straight back as you pull. Brace your chest against the pad. Grip the handle with one hand, and firmly hold the back of the pad with the other.

2 Bend the elbow of your working arm to pull straight back until you are in the fully contracted position. Return to the starting position, and repeat for 8 to 10 repetitions, and then repeat with the opposite arm.

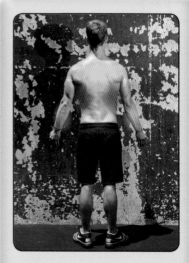

MUSCLE ACTION
Primary activation
- latissimus dorsi
- outer back

Ancillary activation
- biceps brachii
- rear deltoids
- rhomboids
- wrist and forearm flexors
- wrist and forearm extensors

PROPER FORM
Do
- Maintain a flat back throughout the movement.
- Move through a full and controlled range of motion.
- Contract each repetition at the top of the movement.

Avoid
- Rounding your back.
- Twisting your torso.
- Letting the weight swing back following the completion of each repetition.

MODIFICATIONS
Beginner
- Use a lighter weight.

Advanced
- Alternate arms.

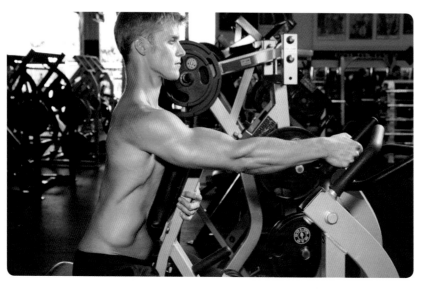

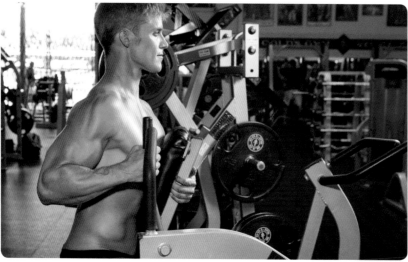

SINGLE-ARM LOW ROW

PROGRESSION

1 Begin by leaning forward while maintaining a flat back with slightly bent legs and holding the handle of a single pulley in one hand with your palm facing inward.

2 Pull the handle back and close to your chest, feeling the contraction in your lats.

3 Lower, and repeat for 8 to 10 repetitions, and then repeat with the opposite arm.

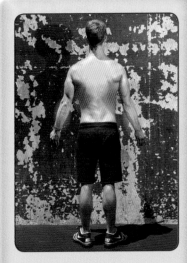

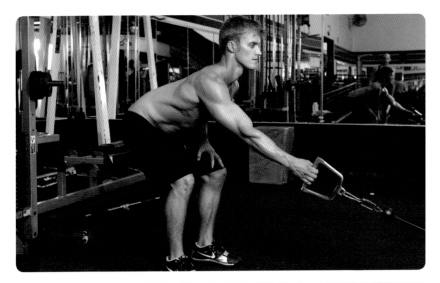

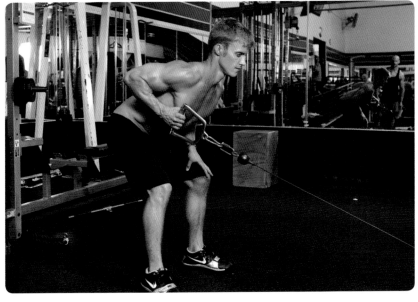

MUSCLE ACTION
Primary activation
- latissimus dorsi
- outer back

Ancillary activation
- biceps brachii
- rear deltoids
- rhomboids
- wrist and forearm flexors
- wrist and forearm extensors

PROPER FORM
Do
- Maintain a flat back throughout the movement.
- Move through a full and controlled range of motion.
- Contract each repetition at the top of the movement.

Avoid
- Rounding your back.
- Twisting your torso.
- Letting the cable stack drop following the completion of each repetition.

MODIFICATIONS
Beginner
- Use a rope or cable attachment with two handles.

Advanced
- Raise one leg.

KETTLEBELL ONE-ARM ROW

PROGRESSION

1 Begin in a standing, staggered stance, holding a kettlebell in the hand on the same side as the back foot. Bend forward at the waist while maintaining a flat back, and then place one hand on your front thigh and allow the working arm to hang straight downward.

2 Bend your elbow back to row the kettlebell in toward your abdomen.

3 Lower back to full extension, and then repeat for 8 to 10 repetitions.

4 Repeat with the opposite arm.

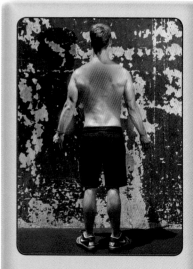

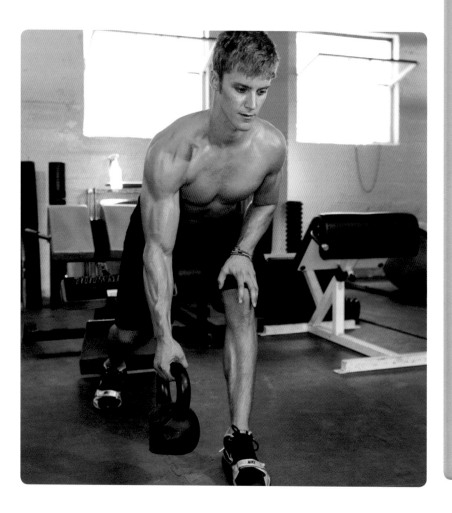

MUSCLE ACTION

Primary activation
- latissimus dorsi
- rhomboids
- trapezius

Ancillary activation
- biceps
- posterior deltoids
- wrist and forearm flexors
- wrist and forearm extensors

PROPER FORM

Do
- Maintain a flat back throughout the movement.
- Pull both back and up.
- Contract your back at the top of the movement.

Avoid
- Rounding your back.
- Excessively swinging the kettlebell.
- Allowing the kettlebell to drop following the completion of each repetition.

MODIFICATIONS

Beginner
- Use a lighter weight.

Advanced
- Use both arms simultaneously.

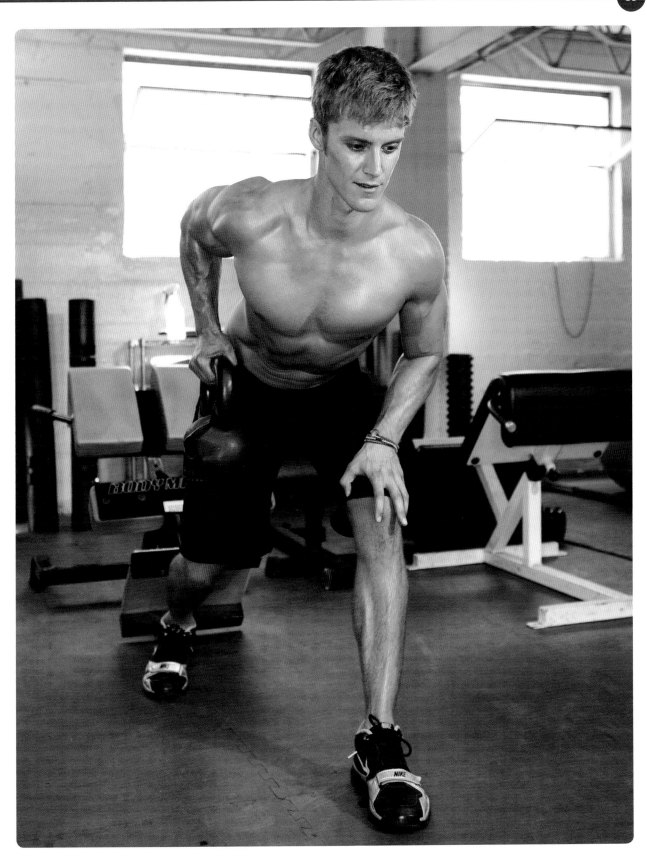

MACHINE PULLOVER

PROGRESSION

1 Begin seated in a pullover machine. Adjust the seat so that when your arms are raised overhead, your elbows will be centered on the elbow pads.

2 Step on the bar at your feet to bring the apparatus in front of you. Place your elbows on the pad, and grasp the bar with an overhand grip, and then step off the bar. Stretch your arms backward to the start position.

3 Drive your elbows down and back so that the bar moves toward your abdomen, contracting your latissimus dorsi muscles as you move.

4 Stretch back, and perform 8 to 10 repetitions. When finished, use the foot bar to catch the weight, and then remove your arms and slowly let the weight fall.

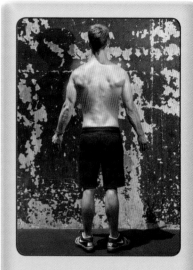

MUSCLE ACTION
Primary activation
- latissimus dorsi
- serratus anterior

Ancillary activation
- deltoids
- triceps brachii
- rectus abdominis

PROPER FORM
Do
- Lower the bar with control.
- Fully expand your chest.
- Keep your elbows firmly on the pads throughout the exercise.

Avoid
- Pulling away from the back pad.
- Excessively stretching behind your head.
- Releasing your arms from the bar before pushing the foot bar.

MODIFICATIONS
Beginner
- Use a lighter weight.

Advanced
- Use a closer, underhand grip.

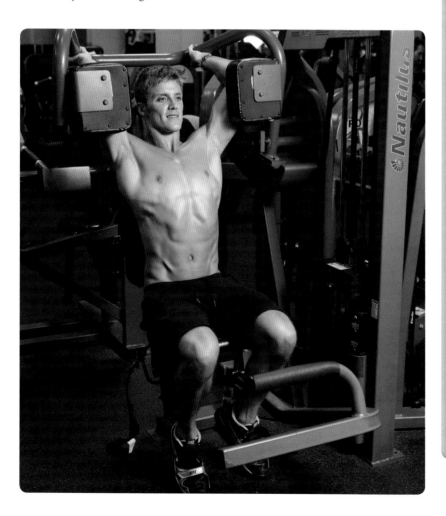

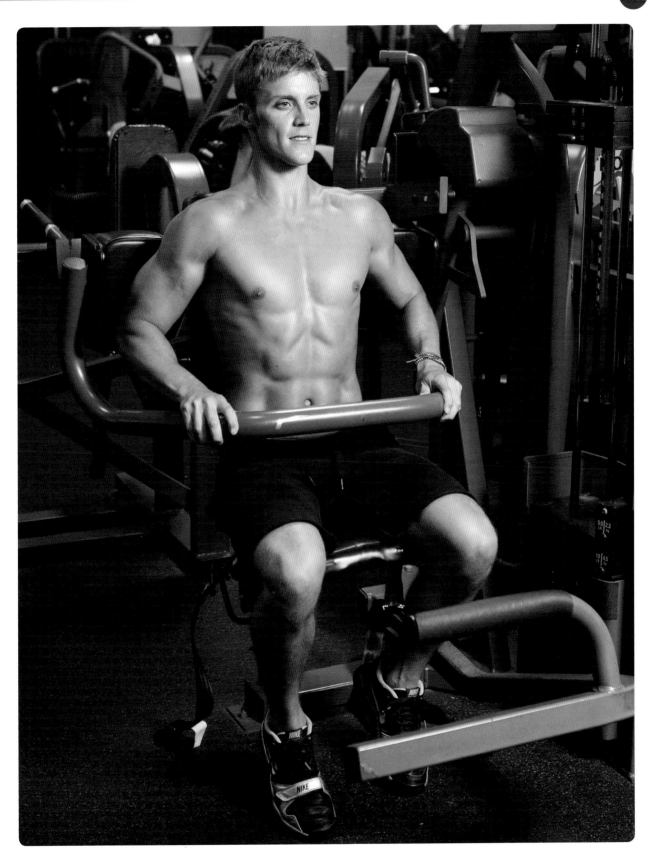

REVERSE-GRIP PULLDOWN

PROGRESSION

1 Begin seated at a pulldown machine while maintaining a close, underhand grip on the bar.

2 Pull the bar down to the very top of your chest, contracting your lats, and then slowly extend the bar back up to full extension. Perform 8 to 10 repetitions.

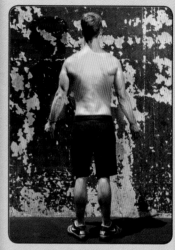

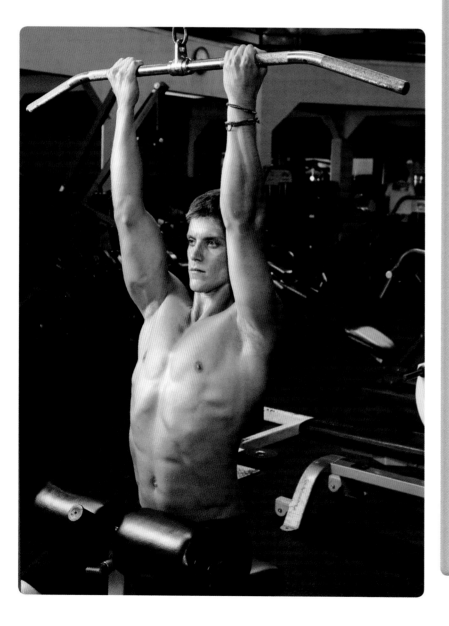

MUSCLE ACTION
Primary activation
- latissimus dorsi

Ancillary activation
- anterior deltoids
- trapezius
- rhomboids
- biceps brachii
- wrist and forearm flexors
- wrist and forearm extensors

PROPER FORM
Do
- Move through a full and controlled range of motion.
- Lower your shoulders in the completed movement.
- Maintain a flat back throughout the movement.

Avoid
- Overarching your back.
- Excessively swinging the weight.
- Pulling the bar too far below your chest.

MODIFICATIONS
Beginner
- Use a wider grip to decrease range of motion.

Advanced
- Use an overhand grip.

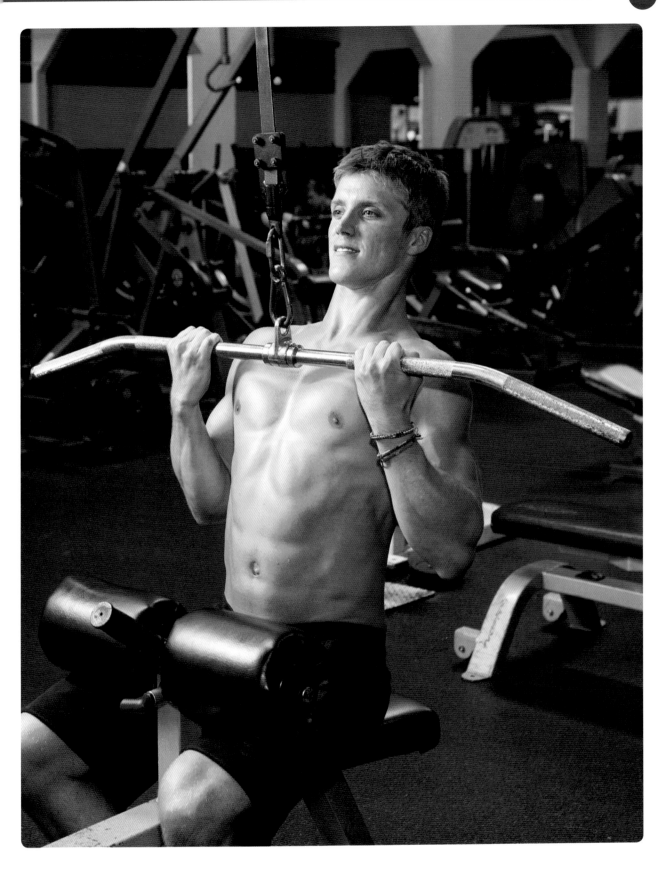

PULL-UP

PROGRESSION

1 Begin by standing in front of a pull-up bar and take an overhand, shoulder-width grip and hang below at arm's length.

2 Pull yourself up, contracting your lats at the peak position, and then lower to arm's length. Perform 8 to 10 repetitions.

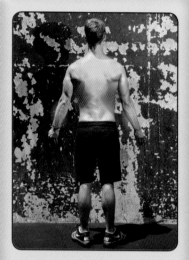

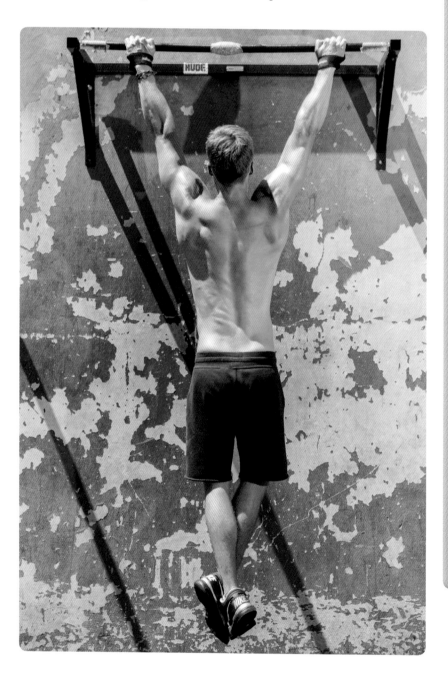

MUSCLE ACTION
Primary activation
• latissimus dorsi

Ancillary activation
• biceps brachii
• trapezius
• rhomboids
• wrist and forearm flexors
• wrist and forearm extensors

PROPER FORM
Do
• Lower yourself with control.
• Pull your chin toward the bar.
• Contract your lats at the top of the movement.

Avoid
• Pulling behind your neck.
• Excessive body swinging.
• Using your arms instead of your lats to lift yourself.

MODIFICATIONS
Beginner
• Have someone assist you at your legs.

Advanced
• Grip a dumbbell between your lower legs.

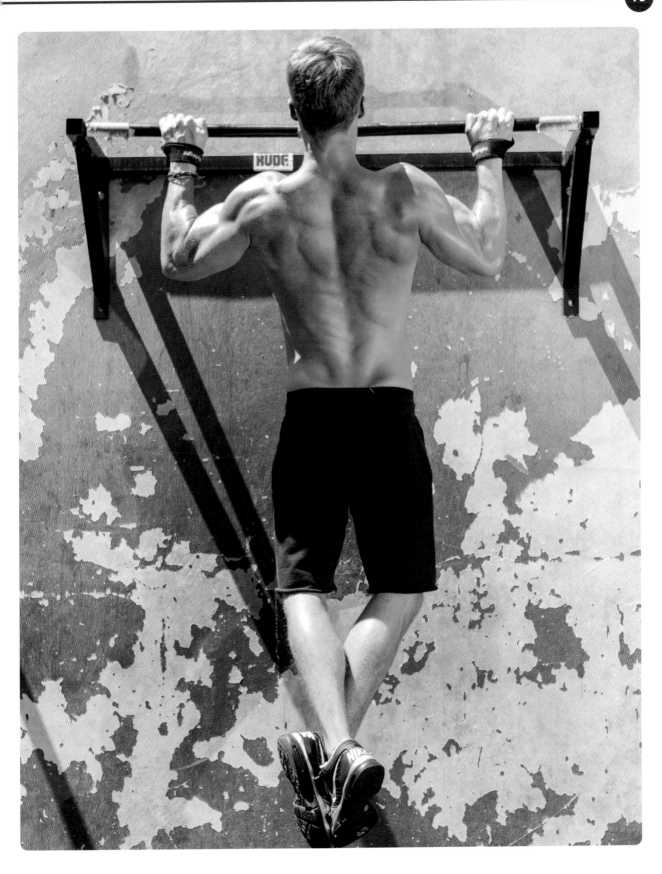

INCLINE DUMBBELL PRESS

PROGRESSION

1 Begin by lying back on an incline bench with your feet planted on the ground. With a dumbbell in each hand, position them at the sides of your chest with your upper arm under each dumbbell.

2 Start by extending your arms upward to full extension over your upper chest.

3 Lower down the same pathway for 6 to 10 repetitions.

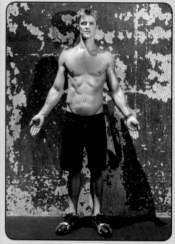

MUSCLE ACTION
Primary activation
- pectoralis major

Ancillary activation
- anterior deltoids
- triceps brachii
- rectus abdominis
- erector spinae

PROPER FORM
Do
- Use a controlled descent.
- Bring the dumbbells to your outer shoulders.
- Keep your feet planted on the ground.

Avoid
- Arching your back.
- Bouncing the dumbbells off your chest.
- Excessive speed.

MODIFICATIONS
Beginner
- Reduce the angle of incline.

Advanced
- Alternate arms.

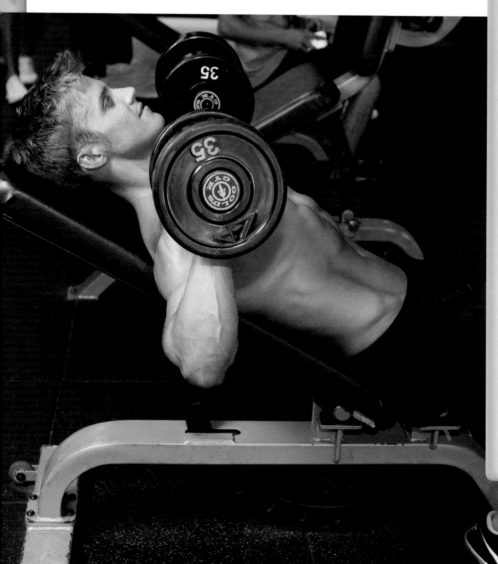

CHEST TIPS
For some, the pectorals, or chest muscles, can be difficult to control while training. In order to feel the pectoral muscles contract, stretch one arm out to the side and place your other hand on that side's chest. Slowly draw the arm across your torso while keeping your arm straight, and you will feel a contraction. It is important not to get caught up in how much weight you are lifting, but instead concentrate on how much you can feel the muscles contract during the execution of the movement.

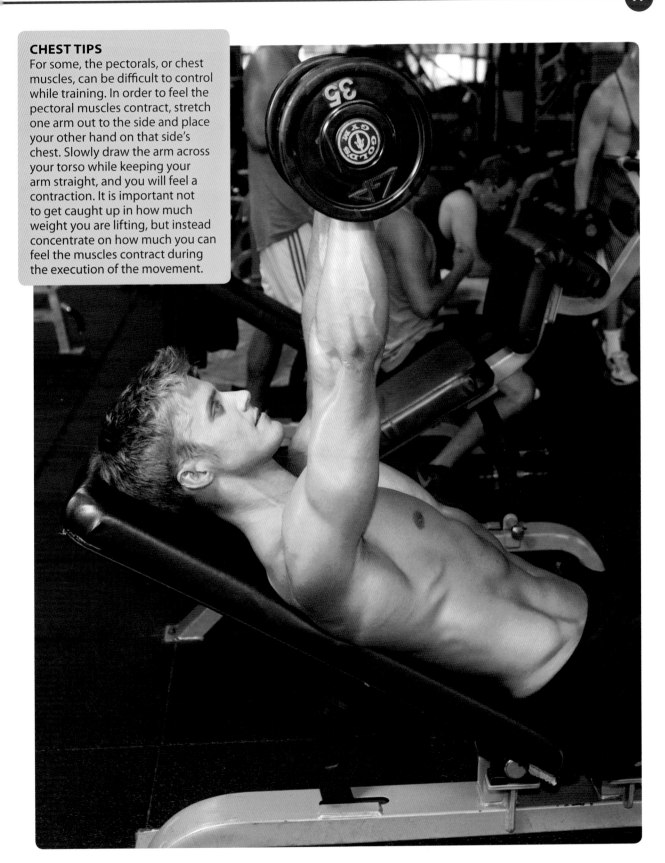

HAMMER STRENGTH INCLINE PRESS

PROGRESSION

1 Begin seated in a Hammer Strength machine with your feet planted on the ground and your hands on the grips in line with your shoulders.

2 Extend your arms upward to full extension until your chest is in the fully contracted position.

3 Return to the starting position for 8 to 10 repetitions.

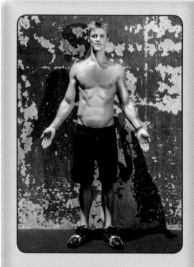

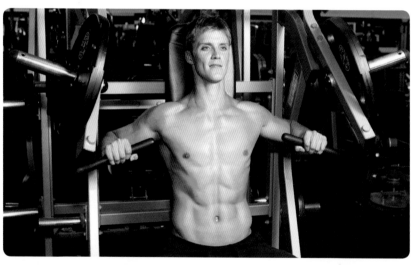

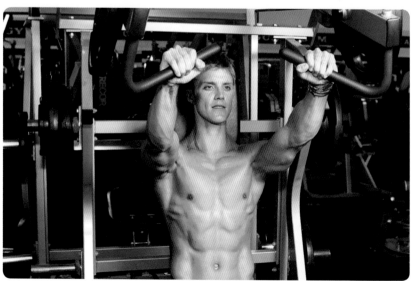

MUSCLE ACTION
Primary activation
• pectoralis major

Ancillary activation
• anterior deltoids
• triceps brachii
• rectus abdominis
• erector spinae

PROPER FORM
Do
• Achieve a full extension.
• Lower with control.
• Keep your hands in line with your shoulders.

Avoid
• Bouncy or partial repetitions.
• A fast or sloppy descent.
• Allowing your lower back to move away from the pad.

MODIFICATIONS
Beginner
• Use a wider grip to decrease range of motion.

Advanced
• Alternate arms.

FLAT BARBELL PRESS

PROGRESSION

1 Begin lying back on a flat bench with your feet planted on the ground and a shoulder-width grip on the bar.

2 Start by lowering the barbell to your nipple line.

3 Push back up to full extension for 6 to 10 repetitions.

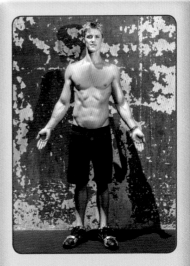

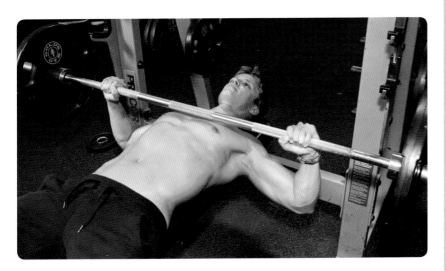

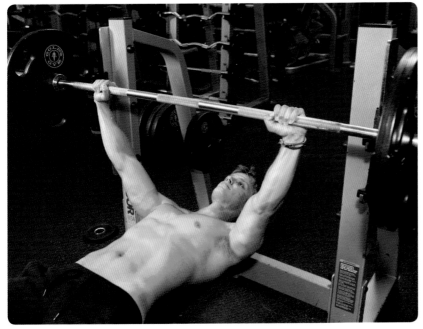

MUSCLE ACTION
Primary activation
- pectoralis major

Ancillary activation
- anterior deltoids
- triceps brachii
- rectus abdominis
- erector spinae

PROPER FORM
Do
- Use a controlled descent.
- Lower the barbell to your nipple line.
- Keep your feet planted on the ground.

Avoid
- Arching your back.
- Bouncing the bar off your chest.
- Excessive speed.

MODIFICATIONS
Beginner
- Use a wider grip to decrease range of motion.

Advanced
- Use a closer grip to increase range of motion.

FLAT DUMBBELL FLY

PROGRESSION

1 Begin by lying back on a flat bench with your feet planted on the ground and two dumbbells locked out directly over your chest with your palms facing each other.

2 Forming an arc, lower the dumbbells to the sides until your chest muscles are stretched with your elbows fixed in a slightly bent position.

3 With a hugging motion, bring the dumbbells together until they nearly touch, lengthening your arms as you move. Perform 8 to 10 controlled repetitions.

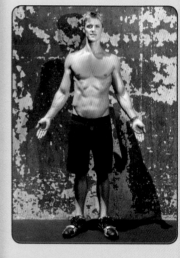

MUSCLE ACTION
Primary activation
• pectoralis major

Ancillary activation
• anterior deltoids
• rectus abdominis
• erector spinae

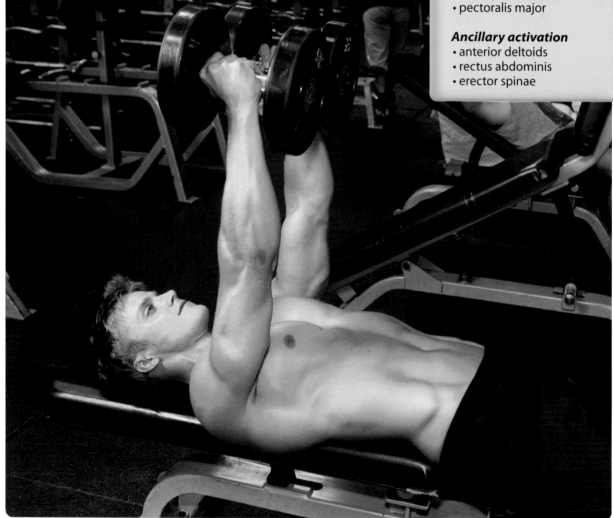

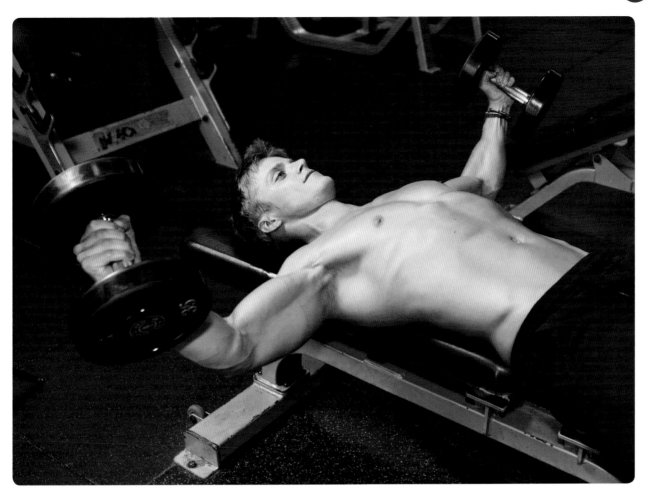

PROPER FORM
Do
- Lower the dumbbells with control.
- Squeeze your pecs together at the top of the movement.
- Keep your arms slightly bent during the outward phase.

Avoid
- Arching your back.
- Straightening your arms out to your sides.
- Excessive speed.

MODIFICATIONS
Beginner
- Use a lighter weight.

Advanced
- Alternate arms.

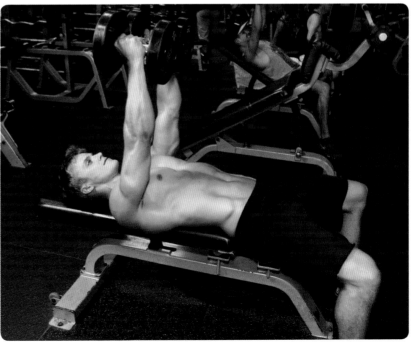

CABLE CROSSOVER

PROGRESSION

1 Begin standing in the middle of a pulley stack with the cables set at the high position, one handle in each hand, with a staggered stance.

2 Lean forward, and bend your arms as you draw them across your chest until your knuckles are nearly touching.

3 Contract your chest, then return your arms to the outstretched position in a controlled manner, and repeat for 10 to 12 repetitions.

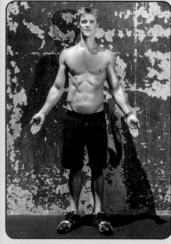

MUSCLE ACTION
Primary activation
• pectoralis major

Ancillary activation
• anterior deltoids
• rhomboids
• rectus abdominis

PROPER FORM
Do
• Look for a controlled lengthening of the arms.
• Keep your torso stabilized.
• Maintain a huglike motion throughout the exercise.

Avoid
• Excessive speed.
• Relying too much on anterior deltoids.
• Leaning too far forward.

MODIFICATIONS
Beginner
• Use a lighter weight.

Advanced
• Alternate arms.

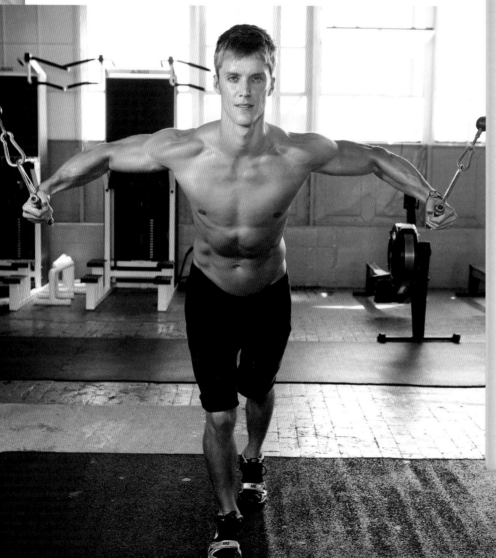

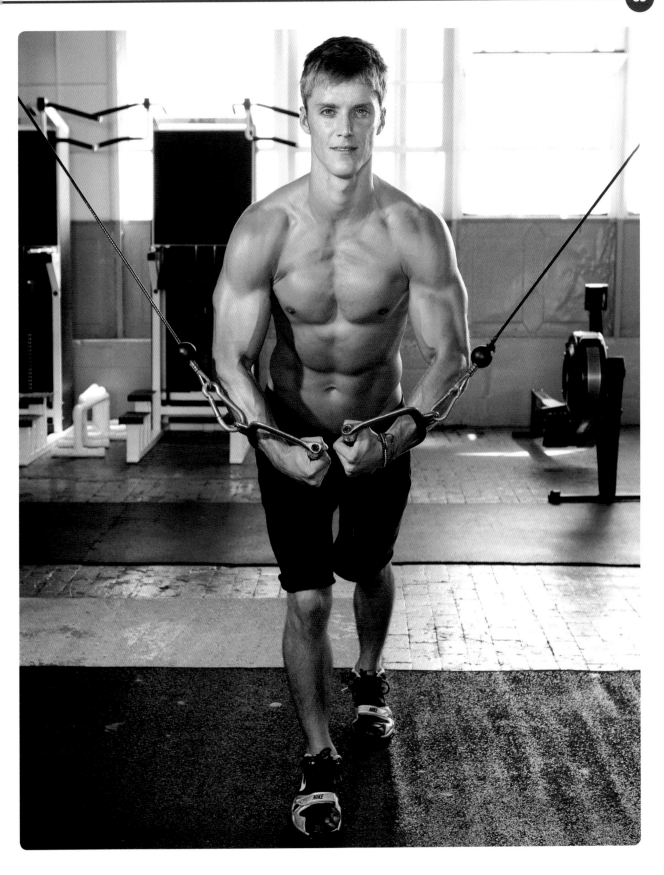

EZ-CURL BARBELL CURL

PROGRESSION

1 Begin by standing with your arms fully extended holding an EZ-curl barbell with an underhand, shoulder-width grip.

2 Bend your arms, curling the barbell upward, until your hands are nearly touching your shoulders.

3 Return the barbell downward to the starting position, and repeat for 8 to 10 repetitions.

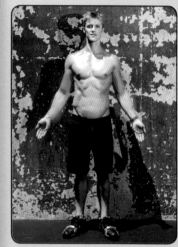

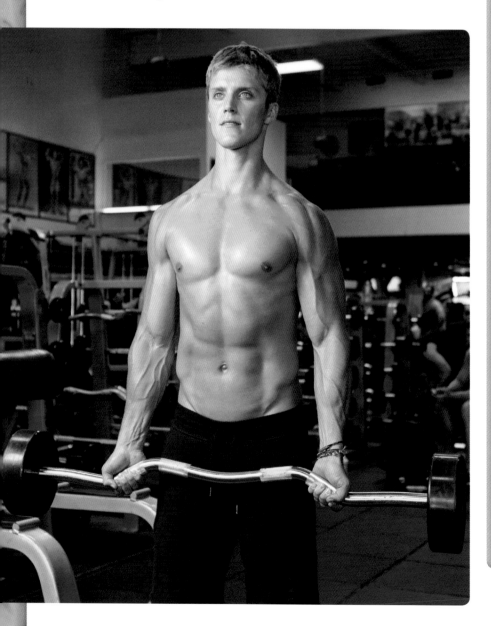

MUSCLE ACTION
Primary activation
• biceps brachii

Ancillary activation
• wrist and forearm flexors
• wrist and forearm extensors
• rectus abdominis
• erector spinae

PROPER FORM
Do
• Move through a full and controlled range of motion.
• Keep your elbows close to your body throughout the movement.
• Lower the bar with control.

Avoid
• Using momentum to swing the weight up.
• Speedy repetitions.
• Excessively using your lower-back muscles.

MODIFICATIONS
Beginner
• Use a wider grip to decrease range of motion.

Advanced
• Use a closer grip to increase range of motion.

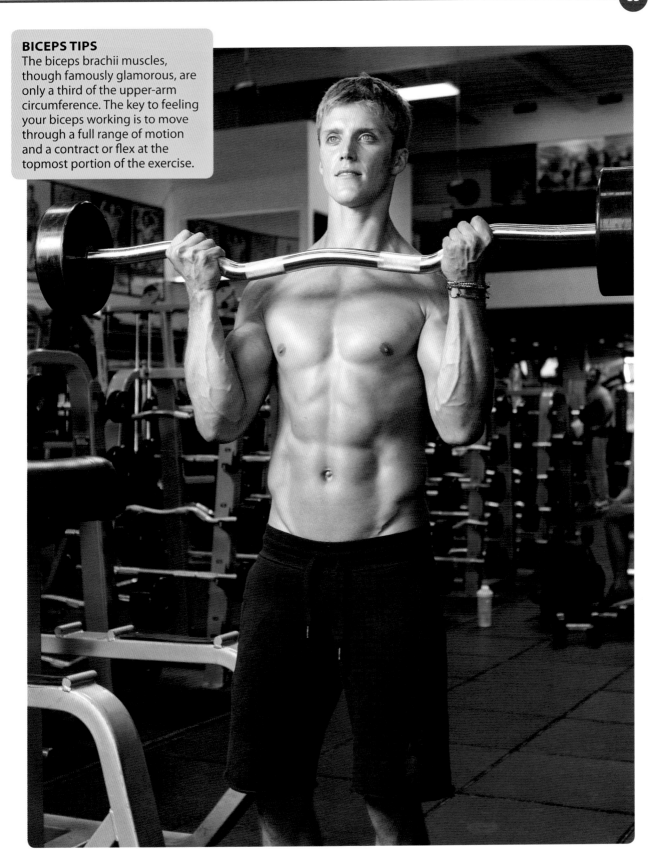

BICEPS TIPS
The biceps brachii muscles, though famously glamorous, are only a third of the upper-arm circumference. The key to feeling your biceps working is to move through a full range of motion and a contract or flex at the topmost portion of the exercise.

ALTERNATE HAMMER CURL

PROGRESSION

1 Begin by standing with your arms fully extended holding a pair of dumbbells with your palms facing each other.

2 Bend one arm at the elbow and curl the dumbbell upward until your hand nearly touches your shoulders.

3 Return downward to the starting position, and repeat with the other arm. Continue alternating arms for 8 to 10 repetitions per side.

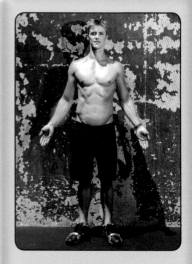

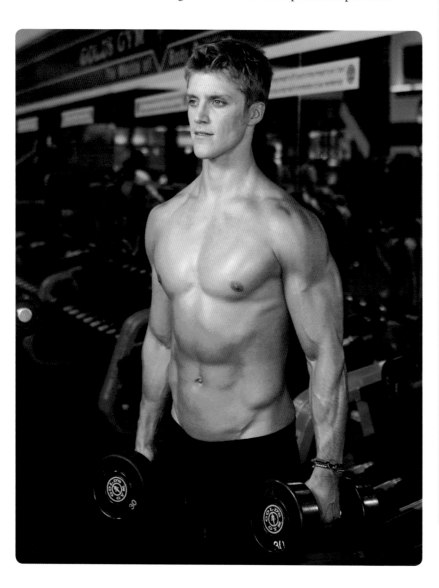

MUSCLE ACTION
Primary activation
- biceps brachii
- brachialis

Ancillary activation
- wrist and forearm flexors
- wrist and forearm extensors
- rectus abdominis
- erector spinae

PROPER FORM
Do
- Point your thumbs upward throughout the movement.
- Keep your elbows close to your body.
- Lower the dumbbells with control.

Avoid
- Using momentum to swing the weight up.
- Speedy repetitions.
- Excessively using your lower-back muscles.

MODIFICATIONS
Beginner
- Use a lighter weight.

Advanced
- Use both arms simultaneously.

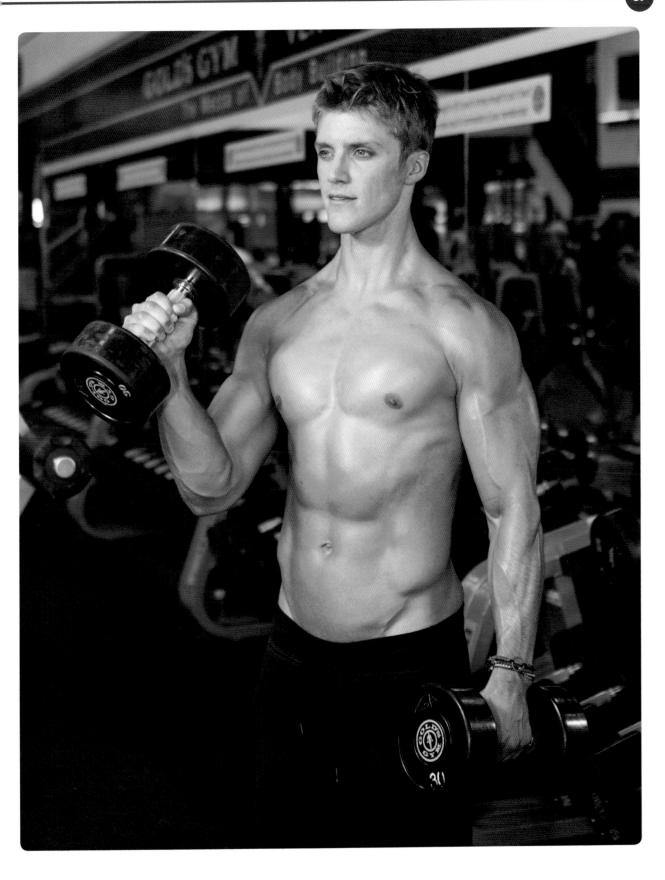

PREACHER CURL

PROGRESSION

1 Begin seated at a preacher bench with your arms fully extended holding an EZ-curl barbell with an underhand, shoulder-width grip.

2 Bend your arms, curling the barbell upward, until your hands are nearly touching your shoulders.

3 Return the barbell downward to the starting position, and repeat for 10 to 12 repetitions.

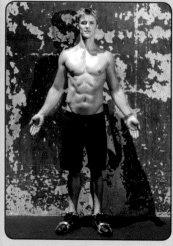

MUSCLE ACTION
Primary activation
- biceps brachii

Ancillary activation
- wrist and forearm flexors
- wrist and forearm extensors

PROPER FORM
Do
- Move through a full and controlled range of motion.
- Keep your elbows in.
- Lower the bar with control.

Avoid
- Allowing your upper arms to lift off the bench.
- Speedy repetitions.
- Using momentum to drive the upward movement of the weight.

MODIFICATIONS
Beginner
- Use a wider grip to decrease range of motion.

Advanced
- Use dumbbells.

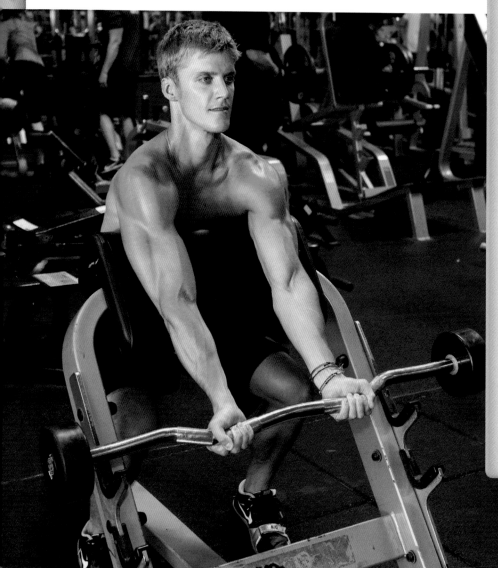

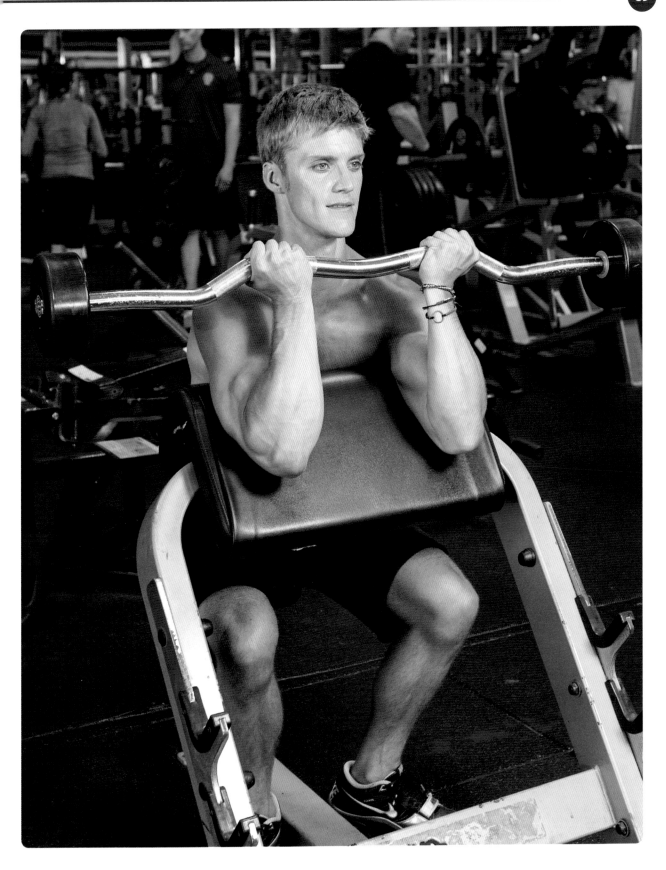

INCLINE DUMBBELL CURL

PROGRESSION

1 Begin by lying back on an incline bench with your feet planted on the ground holding a pair of dumbbells down at your sides with your palms facing one another. Elevate your head.

2 Simultaneously bend your arms at the elbows and turn your wrists upward, curling until your palms are facing upward and nearly touching your shoulders.

3 Return to the starting position by lengthening your arms as you turn your palms outward. Complete 10 to 12 repetitions.

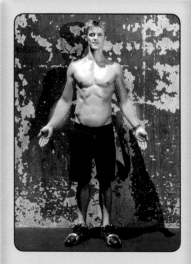

MUSCLE ACTION
Primary activation
• biceps brachii

Ancillary activation
• wrist and forearm flexors
• wrist and forearm extensors
• rectus abdominis
• erector spinae

PROPER FORM
Do
• Move through a full and controlled range of motion.
• Keep your back pressed against the pad.
• Lower the dumbbells with control.

Avoid
• Swinging the weight up.
• Speedy repetitions.
• Using momentum to drive the upward movement of the weight.

MODIFICATIONS
Beginner
• Use one arm at a time.

Advanced
• Do not rotate your palms.

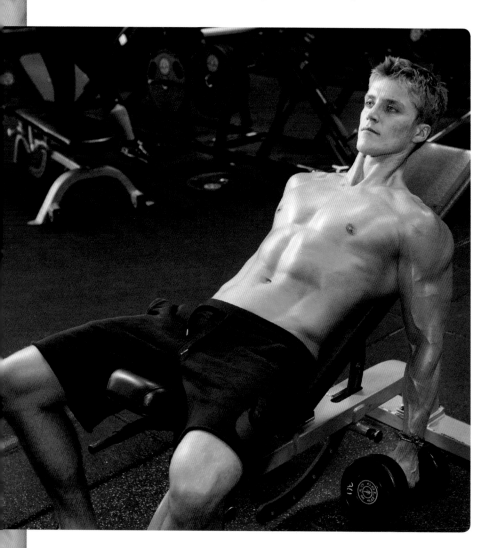

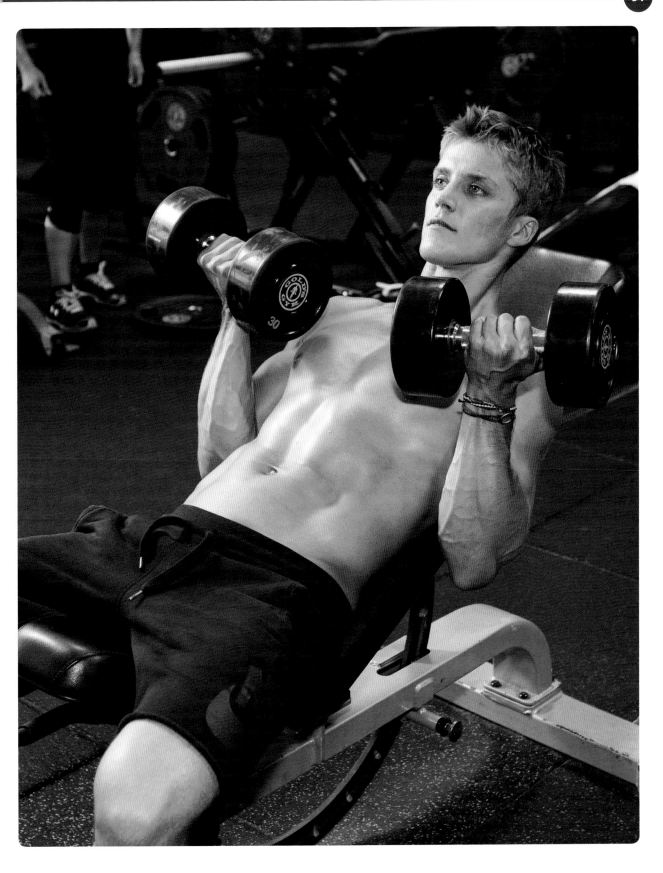

BARBELL SQUAT

PROGRESSION

1 Begin standing in front of a squat rack. Duck under the bar, unracking the barbell and resting it on the rear of your shoulders.

2 Bend your knees slightly, sticking your rear out while keeping your back flat and lowering yourself toward the ground until your thighs are parallel to it.

3 Push through your heels to rise back up, and then repeat for 10 to 12 repetitions.

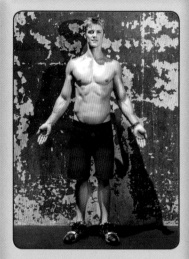

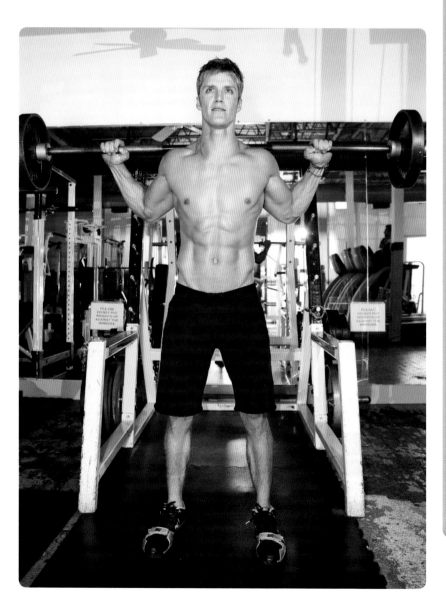

MUSCLE ACTION
Primary activation
- rectus femoris
- vastus lateralis
- vastus intermedius
- vastus medialis
- gluteus maximus
- biceps femoris
- semitendinosus
- semimembranosus

Ancillary activation
- erector spinae
- rectus abdominis
- adductor magnus
- soleus
- gastrocnemius

PROPER FORM
Do
- Squat until your thighs are parallel to the ground.
- Move through a full and controlled range of motion.
- Push through your heels to drive the movement.

Avoid
- Hyperextending your knees past your feet.
- Descending too quickly.
- Pushing through your toes to drive the movement.

QUADRICEPS TIPS

The quadriceps femoris, made up of the rectus femoris, vastus lateralis, vastus intermedius and vastus medialis, is the large group of muscles that sits at the front of your thigh. Due to the size of the quadriceps, it takes a lot of work to properly break them down for renewed muscle growth. When you exercise the quadriceps, it is important to keep the stress on these muscles, and not on your knee joints. Push through your heels instead of your toes when squatting—this will keep the tension on your quadriceps and glutes, which will save your knees. Wearing a weight belt is also a good idea when you perform squats, but avoid wearing one during a set of leg presses, which can result in injured ribs.

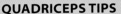

MODIFICATIONS

Beginner
• Use your body weight only.

Advanced
• Take a closer stance to increase range of motion.

REVERSE HACK SQUAT

PROGRESSION

1 Begin standing on the platform of a hack machine with your feet spaced shoulder-width apart, facing the machine so that the pads rest on your shoulders.

2 Rise up to release the weight, and then bend your knees as you lower yourself until your thighs are parallel to the platform.

3 Push through your heels to rise back up. Complete 10 to 12 repetitions.

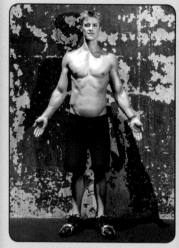

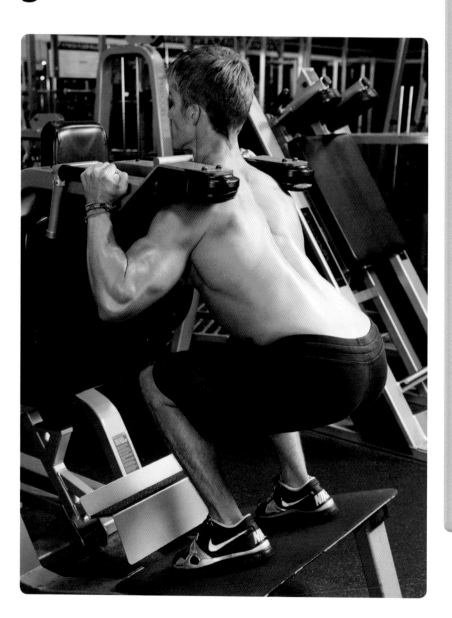

MUSCLE ACTION
Primary activation
- rectus femoris
- vastus lateralis
- vastus intermedius
- vastus medialis
- gluteus maximus
- biceps femoris
- semitendinosus
- semimembranosus

Ancillary activation
- erector spinae
- rectus abdominis
- adductor magnus
- soleus
- gastrocnemius

PROPER FORM
Do
- Squat until your thighs are parallel to the ground.
- Descend slowly with control.
- Push through your heels to drive the movement.

Avoid
- Hyperextending your knees past your feet.
- A partial range of motion.
- Pushing through your toes to drive the movement.

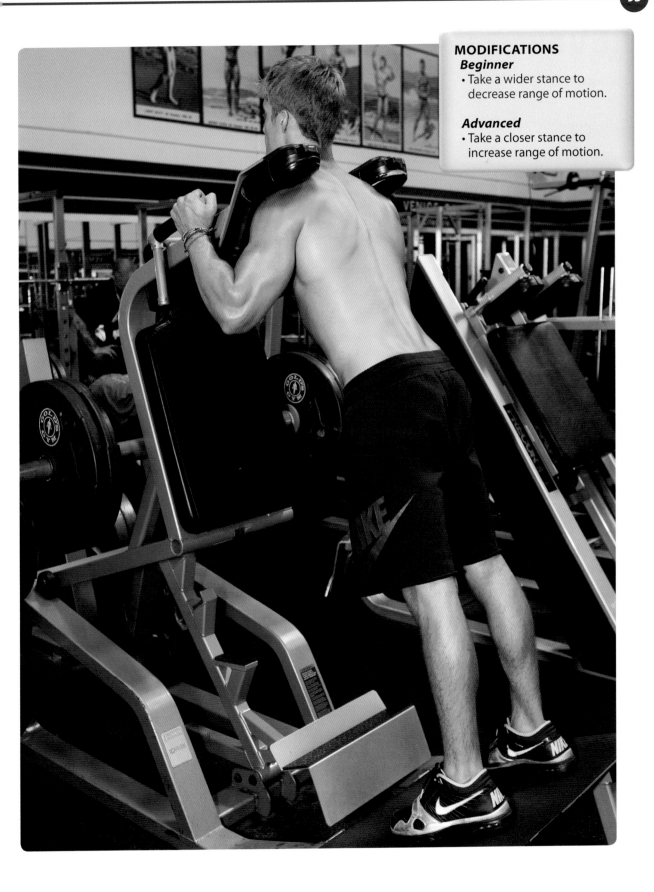

MODIFICATIONS

Beginner
• Take a wider stance to decrease range of motion.

Advanced
• Take a closer stance to increase range of motion.

LEG PRESS

PROGRESSION

1 Begin seated with your back against the pad of a leg press machine and your feet placed less than shoulder-width apart on the foot placement board.

2 Using your hands, unrack the weight as you lower the sled toward your chest.

3 Drive through the heels to a full extension for 10 to 12 repetitions.

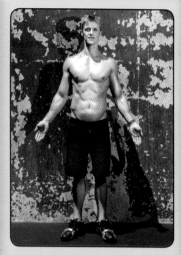

MUSCLE ACTION
Primary activation
- rectus femoris
- vastus lateralis
- vastus intermedius
- vastus medialis
- gluteus maximus
- biceps femoris
- semitendinosus
- semimembranosus

Ancillary activation
- rectus abdominis
- soleus
- gastrocnemius

PROPER FORM
Do
- Push through your heels to drive the movement.
- Lower to roughly a 90-degree angle.
- Exhale as you push up to full extension.

Avoid
- Leading with your toes to drive the movement.
- Lowering too far into your ribcage.
- Allowing your pelvis to raise too high off the seat.

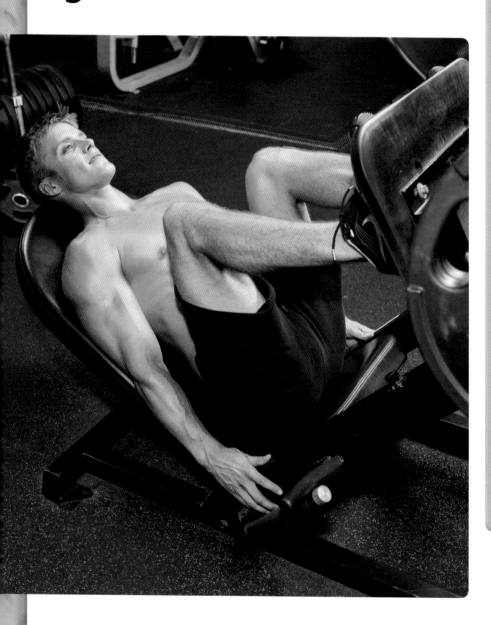

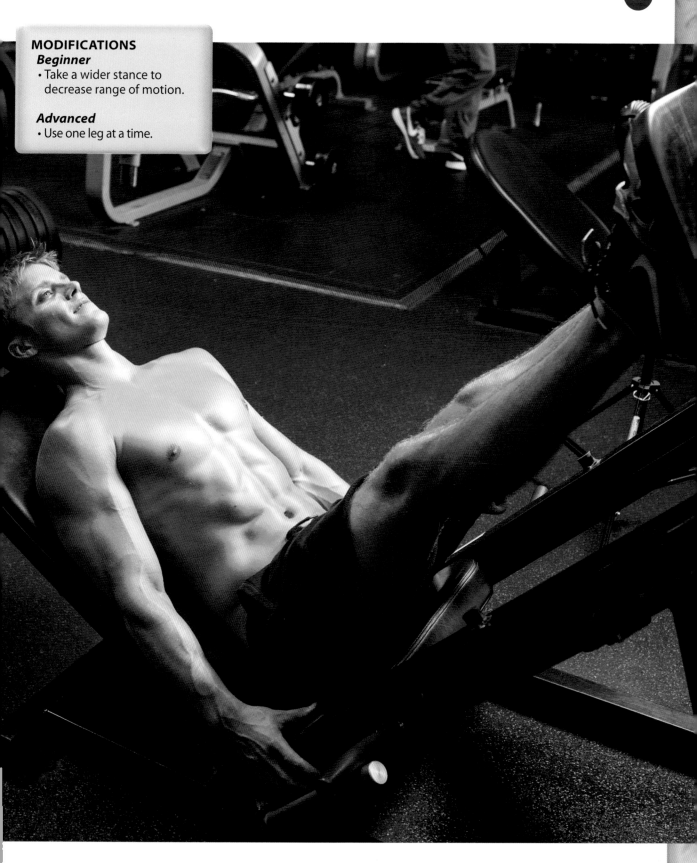

MODIFICATIONS

Beginner
- Take a wider stance to decrease range of motion.

Advanced
- Use one leg at a time.

SMITH MACHINE SPLIT SQUAT

PROGRESSION

1 Begin in a standing position in a Smith machine with the unracked bar placed on the rear of your shoulders. Take a staggered stance with one leg placed forward and one leg placed back.

2 Bend both legs until your front thigh is parallel to the ground and your back heel is elevated.

3 Push through your front heel as you stand to attention, and then lower and repeat for 10 to 12 repetitions per leg.

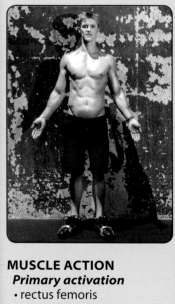

MUSCLE ACTION
Primary activation
- rectus femoris
- vastus lateralis
- vastus intermedius
- vastus medialis
- gluteus maximus
- biceps femoris
- semitendinosus
- semimembranosus

Ancillary activation
- erector spinae
- rectus abdominis
- adductor magnus
- soleus
- gastrocnemius

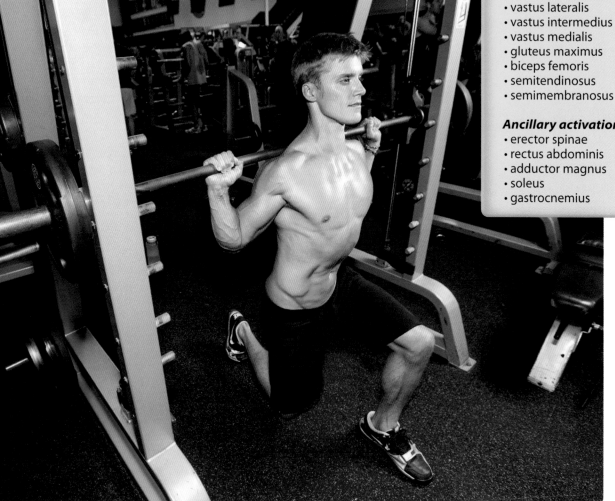

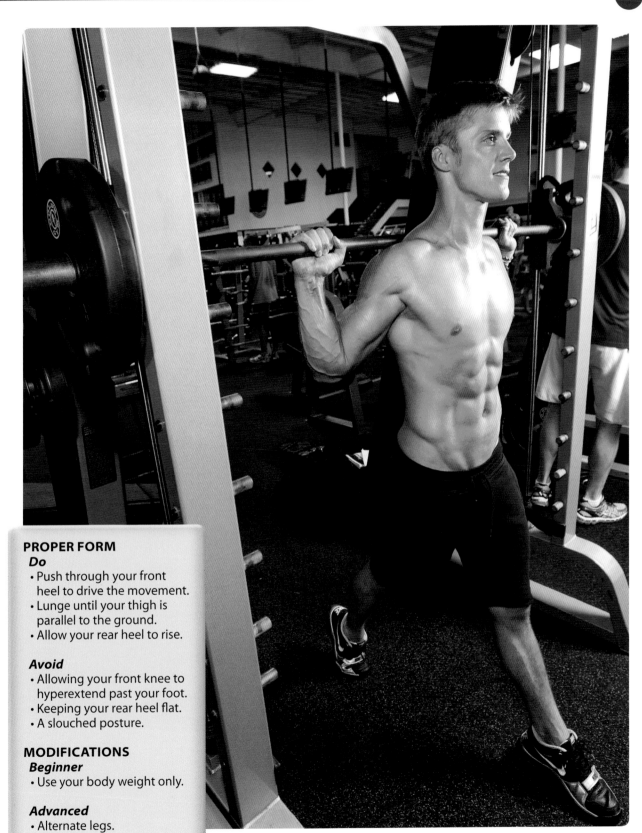

PROPER FORM

Do
- Push through your front heel to drive the movement.
- Lunge until your thigh is parallel to the ground.
- Allow your rear heel to rise.

Avoid
- Allowing your front knee to hyperextend past your foot.
- Keeping your rear heel flat.
- A slouched posture.

MODIFICATIONS

Beginner
- Use your body weight only.

Advanced
- Alternate legs.

LEG EXTENSION
PROGRESSION

1 Begin in a seated position with your back braced against the pad of a leg extension machine and your lower legs placed behind the rollers.

2 Keeping your hands on the grips by your sides, extend your lower legs upward, until your legs are one straight line.

3 Slowly lower back to the starting position, and then repeat for 10 to 12 repetitions.

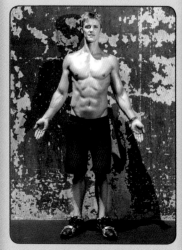

MUSCLE ACTION
Primary activation
- rectus femoris
- vastus lateralis
- vastus intermedius
- vastus medialis

Ancillary activation
- rectus abdominis
- tibialis anterior

PROPER FORM
Do
- Move through a controlled downward range of motion.
- Perform an explosive but controlled positive (raising).
- A peak contraction at the top of the movement.

Avoid
- Speedy or bouncy repetitions.
- Allowing momentum during the repetition.
- Leaning too far forward to cheat the weight up.

MODIFICATIONS
Beginner
- Use a lighter weight.

Advanced
- Try it one leg at a time

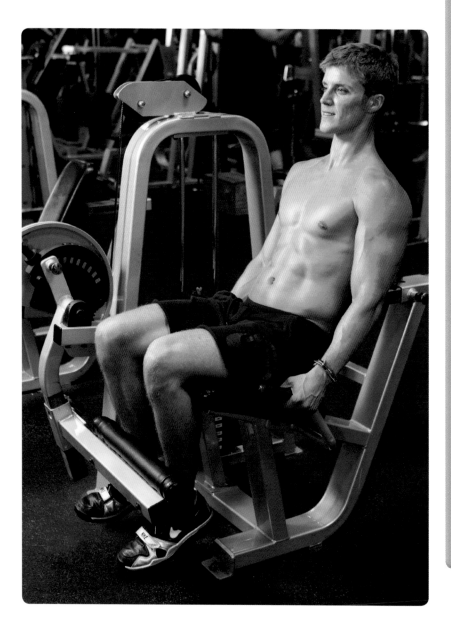

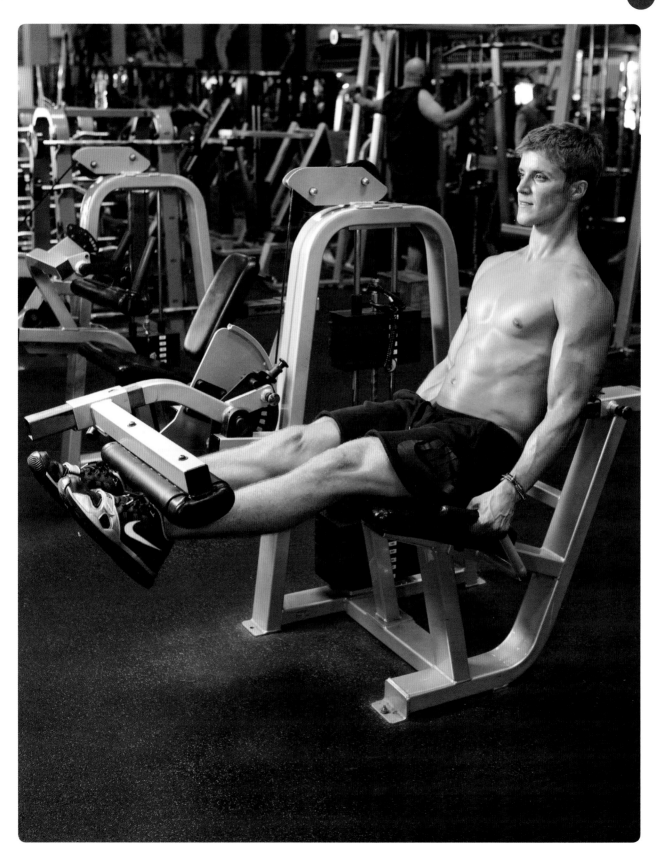

LYING LEG CURL

PROGRESSION

1 Begin lying down on the pad with your lower legs under the rollers, your knees hanging freely, and your hands on the grips.

2 Start by bending your legs back at the knees until fully contracted at the top, nearest the gluteal muscles.

3 Lower back down in a controlled manner to lengthen the muscle, and repeat for 10 to 12 repetitions.

MUSCLE ACTION
Primary activation
- biceps femoris
- semitendinosus
- semimembranosus
- gluteus maximus

Ancillary activation
- gastrocnemius
- erector spinae

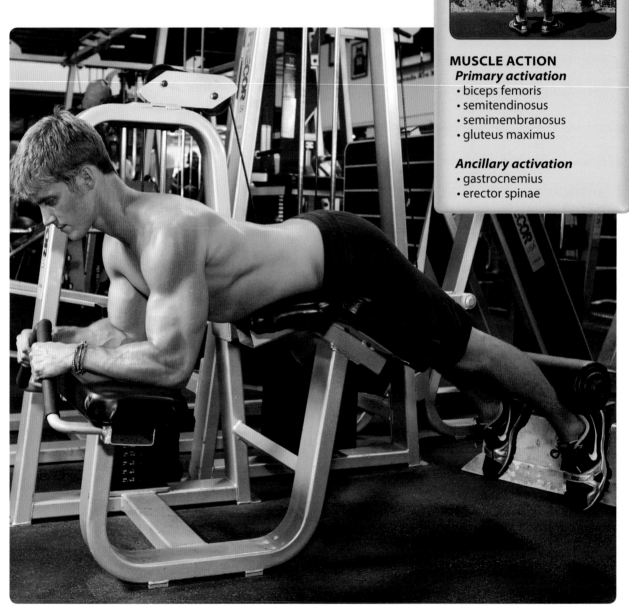

HAMSTRINGS TIPS

The term hamstrings refers to the four tendons contracted by the three muscles at the back of the thigh, but it is also used to refer to the muscles themselves—the biceps femoris, semitendinosus and semimembranosus. Although the dominant quadriceps at the front of the thigh often get the lion's share of attention, the hamstrings are key to maintaining leg flexibility. A good set of hams also fills out the legs not only from the rear, but from the side as well. For maximum stimulation, squeeze the biceps femoris muscle of the leg during exercise as you would the biceps brachii of the upper arm.

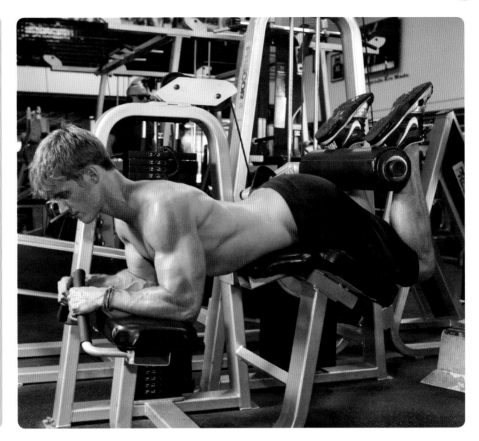

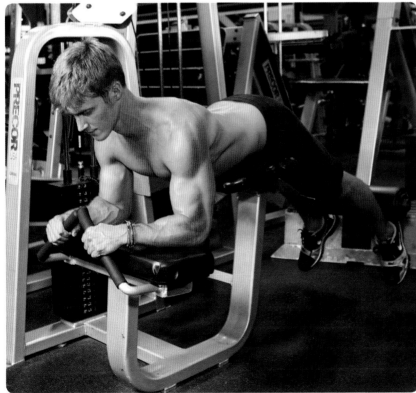

PROPER FORM

Do
- Perform a controlled negative (lowering) and an explosive but controlled positive (raising).
- Contract your hamstrings at the top of the movement.
- Move through a full and controlled range of motion.

Avoid
- Speedy repetitions.
- Using momentum to move the weight up.
- Leaning your upper body backward to cheat the weight up.

MODIFICATIONS

Beginner
- Use a lighter weight.

Advanced
- Use one leg at a time.

SEATED LEG CURL

PROGRESSION

1 Begin seated with your legs extended, your calves resting on the pads of a leg curl machine and your body firmly locked in place.

2 Bend your legs downward and back at the knee until they are fully contracted in the flexed position.

3 Slowly extend your legs back up to the starting position to lengthen the muscle, and repeat for 10 to12 repetitions.

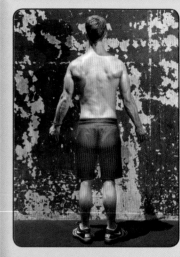

MUSCLE ACTION
Primary activation
- biceps femoris
- semitendinosus
- semimembranosus
- gluteus maximus

Ancillary activation
- gastrocnemius
- gluteus maximus
- rectus abdominis

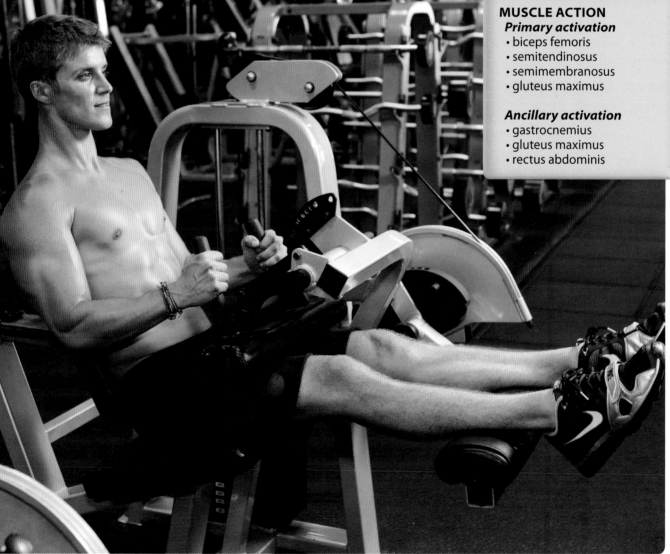

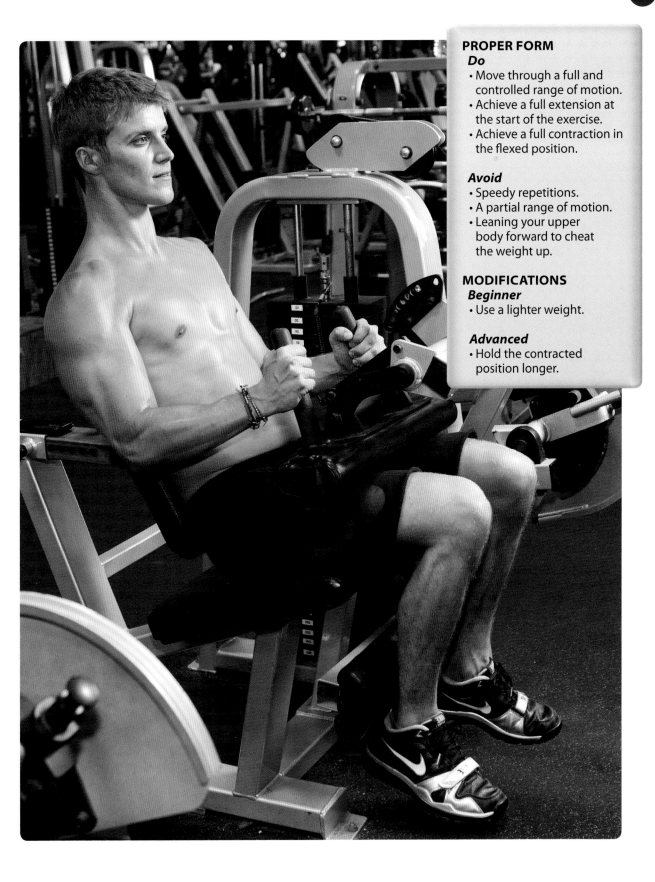

PROPER FORM
Do
- Move through a full and controlled range of motion.
- Achieve a full extension at the start of the exercise.
- Achieve a full contraction in the flexed position.

Avoid
- Speedy repetitions.
- A partial range of motion.
- Leaning your upper body forward to cheat the weight up.

MODIFICATIONS
Beginner
- Use a lighter weight.

Advanced
- Hold the contracted position longer.

STIFF-LEGGED DEADLIFTS

PROGRESSION

1 Begin by holding a barbell with an overhand, shoulder-width grip. Bend your knees slightly, stick your rear out, and while maintaining a flat back, stretch down toward your toes without further bending your legs.

2 Raise up along the same pathway, lifting the barbell no higher than your knees to keep the tension on the targeted muscles. Complete 10 to 12 repetitions.

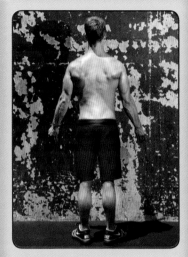

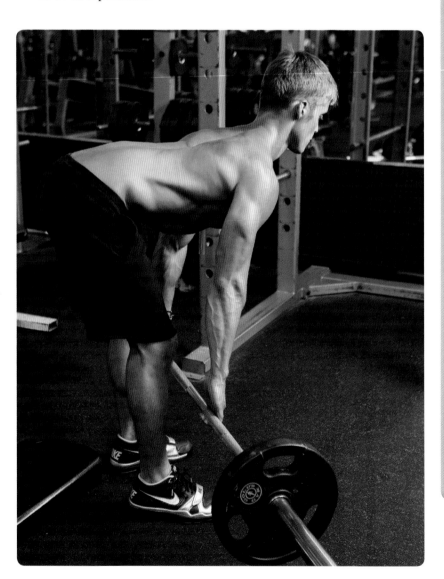

MUSCLE ACTION
Primary activation
- biceps femoris
- semitendinosus
- semimembranosus
- gluteus maximus

Ancillary activation
- gastrocnemius
- erector spinae

PROPER FORM
Do
- Move through a full and controlled range of motion.
- Maintain a flat back throughout the movement.
- Achieve a full extension at the start of the exercise.

Avoid
- Speedy repetitions.
- Completely standing up.
- Rounding your back.

MODIFICATIONS
Beginner
- Use a light pair of dumbbells

Advanced
- Stand on one leg.

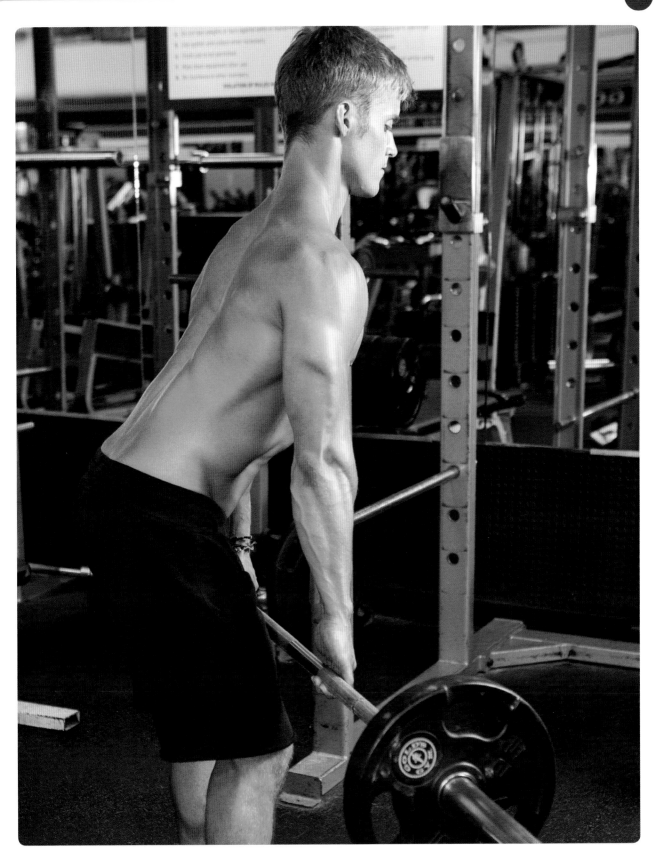

KETTLEBELL STIFF-LEGGED DEADLIFT

PROGRESSION

1 Begin standing with your knees slightly bent and your rear pushed out while holding a kettlebell in front of you. Keep your back flat.

2 Bend forward from your waist, and stretch your hamstrings until the kettlebell is barely touching the ground.

3 Rise back up to a standing position, flexing your glutes and hamstrings, and then lower to repeat for 10 to 12 repetitions.

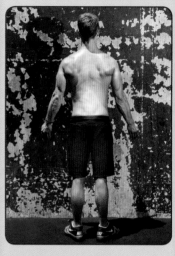

MUSCLE ACTION
Primary activation
- biceps femoris
- semitendinosus
- semimembranosus
- gluteus maximus

Ancillary activation
- gastrocnemius
- erector spinae

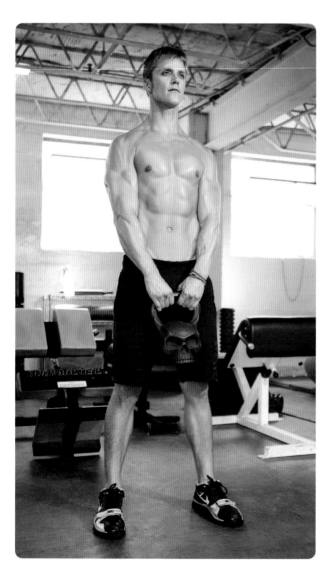

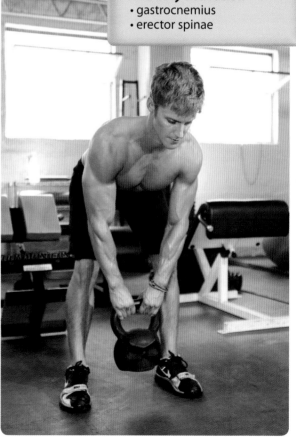

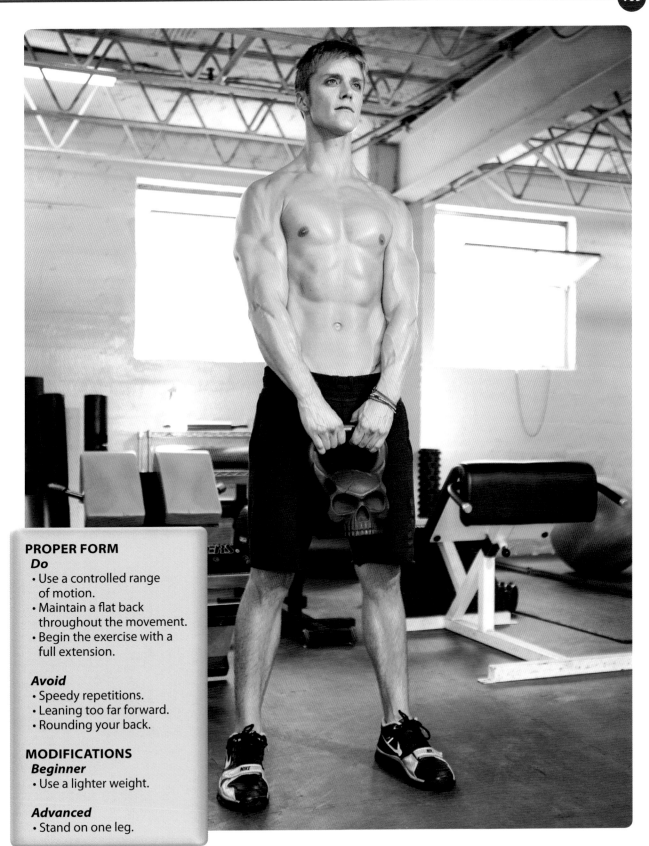

PROPER FORM
Do
- Use a controlled range of motion.
- Maintain a flat back throughout the movement.
- Begin the exercise with a full extension.

Avoid
- Speedy repetitions.
- Leaning too far forward.
- Rounding your back.

MODIFICATIONS
Beginner
- Use a lighter weight.

Advanced
- Stand on one leg.

CALF TIPS

The main calf muscles are the tibialis anterior at the front of the calf and the soleus and gastrocnemius at the back. The tibialis allows you to flex your foot upward and to move your ankle inward. The powerful soleus and gastrocnemius muscles not only complete a set of legs aesthetically, but they also help to literally put the spring in your step and power you through your walking day. Some of us are born with high insertions (making it harder to build), while in others the muscles insert lower, giving the appearance of very long and full calves. Although the shape of your calf is determined by genetics, you can make the most of what you have by properly executing calf exercises. Squeeze each rep at the topmost portion to garner the most benefit from each set, and be sure to move through a full range of motion and stretch during the negative portion of the exercise.

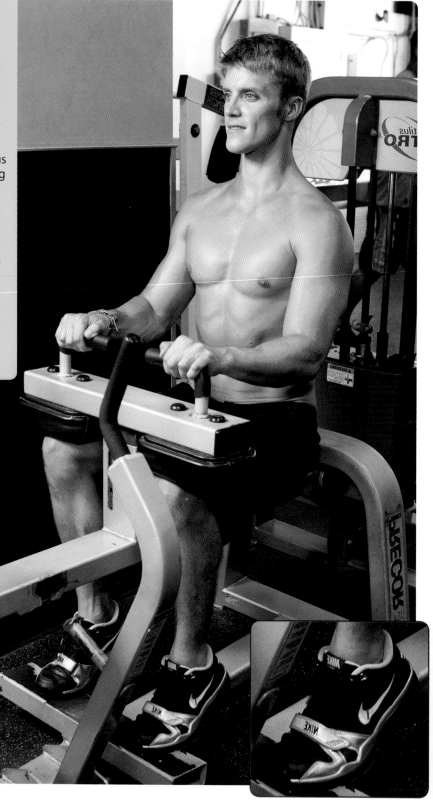

SEATED CALF RAISE

PROGRESSION

1 Begin seated with your thighs under the padding of a calf machine, your toes at the edge of the platform, and your hands on the grips.

2 Raise your heels by extending your ankles as high as possible.

3 Lower your heels past the platform by bending your ankles until your calves are fully stretched. Complete 12 to 15 repetitions.

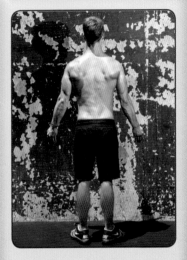

MUSCLE ACTION
Primary activation
- gastrocnemius
- soleus

Ancillary activation
- tibialis anterior

PROPER FORM
Do
- Move through a full and controlled range of motion.
- Contract your calf muscles at the top of the movement.
- Keep your toes pointed straight forward.

Avoid
- Partial repetitions.
- Bouncy or speedy repetitions.
- Having too much of your feet on the platform.

MODIFICATIONS
Beginner
- Use your body weight only.

Advanced
- Point your toes inward to work more of the outer area of your calf muscles.

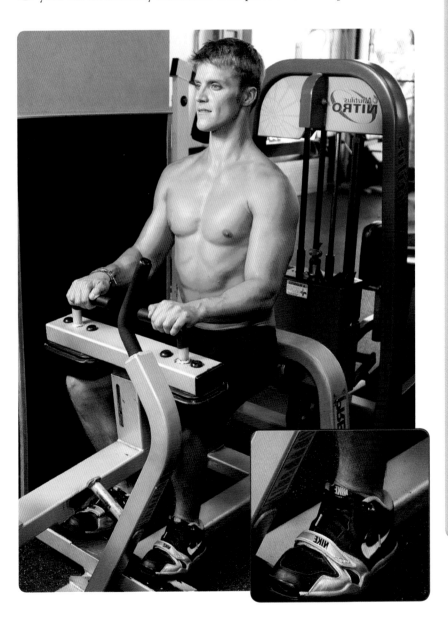

TIBIA RAISE

PROGRESSION

1 Begin seated in a leg press with your back against the pad and your toes placed less than shoulder-width apart on the edge of the foot placement board.

2 Rise up on your toes to contract your calf muscles, and then lower your feet back down to the flat starting position. Complete 12 to 15 repetitions.

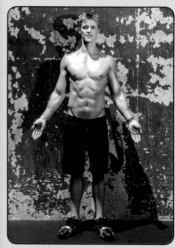

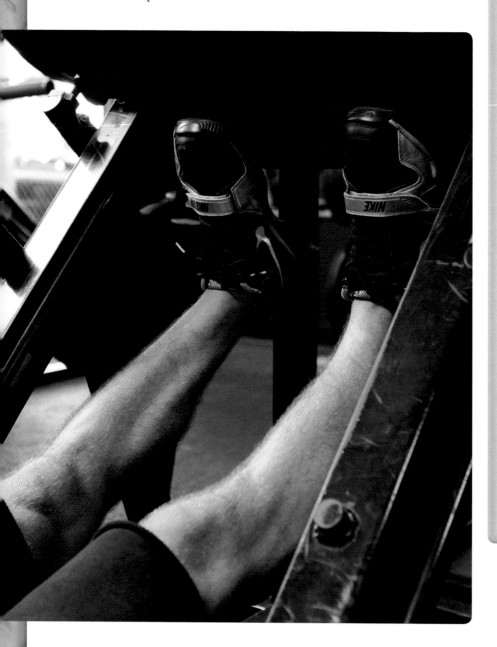

MUSCLE ACTION
Primary activation
- tibialis anterior
- soleus

Ancillary activation
- gastrocnemius

PROPER FORM
Do
- Move through a full and controlled range of motion.
- Contract your calf muscles at the top of the movement.
- Keep your toes pointed straight forward.

Avoid
- Partial repetitions.
- Bouncy or speedy repetitions.
- Having too much of your toes on the platform will limit your range of motion.

MODIFICATIONS
Beginner
- Use a lighter weight.

Advanced
- Use one leg at a time.

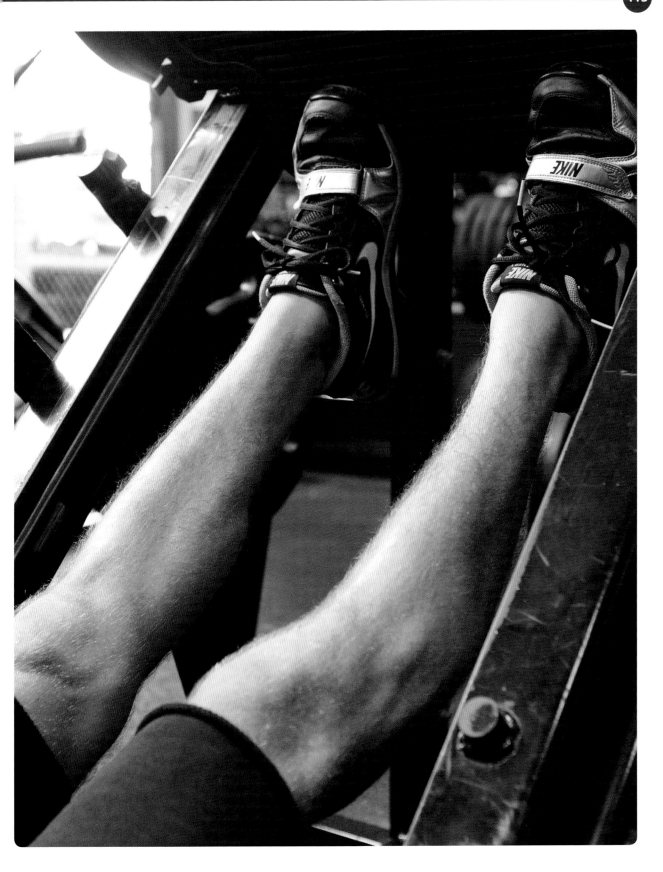

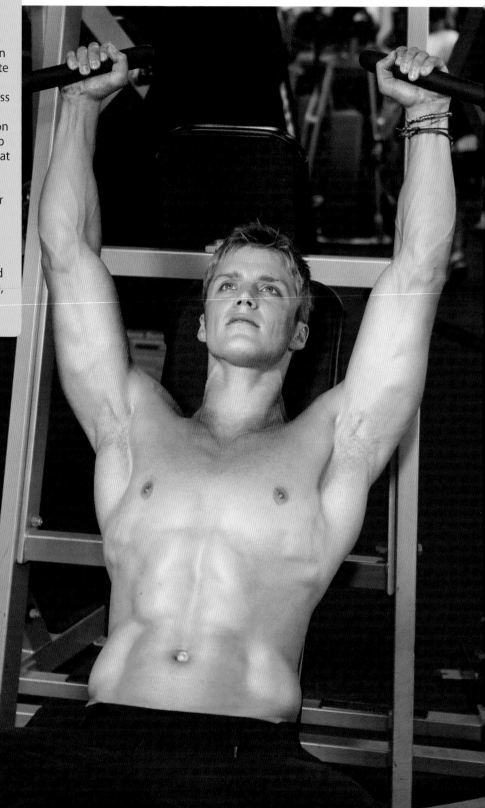

SHOULDER TIPS
The deltoid muscles of the shoulders are responsible for the 360-degree rotation of your arms, and they quite literally cap off your upper body. Never perform a press behind the neck, because this can put undue strain on your rotator cuff, the group of muscles and tendons that stabilize the shoulder. It is also important that when performing lateral raises or flyes to point your thumbs downward as you ascend. This will keep the tension where it belongs on the medial deltoid muscle, and not on the anterior deltoid, which would negate your overall development.

HAMMER STRENGTH SHOULDER PRESS

PROGRESSION

1 Begin in a seated position on the Hammer Strength shoulder press machine while gripping the handles.

2 Press upward to a full extension, and then lower back down the same pathway, and repeat for 6 to 10 repetitions.

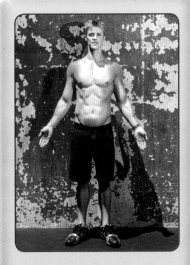

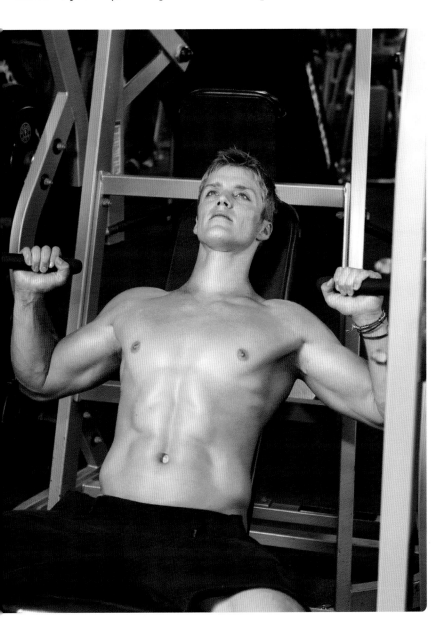

MUSCLE ACTION
Primary activation
- anterior deltoids

Ancillary activation
- lateral deltoids
- triceps brachii
- trapezius
- rhomboids
- rectus abdominis
- erector spinae

PROPER FORM
Do
- Perform slow and controlled repetitions.
- Keep your torso stabilized and your back pressed against the pad.
- Be sure to push overhead.

Avoid
- A partial range of motion.
- Pressing away from your chest as in a chest press.
- Arching your back.

MODIFICATIONS
Beginner
- Use a lighter weight.

Advanced
- Alternate arms.

STANDING MILITARY PRESS

PROGRESSION

1 Begin in a standing position with a staggered stance while holding a barbell with a wide, overhand grip just above your upper chest.

2 Push the bar directly overhead to a full lockout while maintaining an erect posture.

3 Reverse, and return to the starting position for 6 to 8 repetitions.

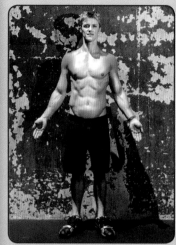

MUSCLE ACTION
Primary activation
• anterior deltoids

Ancillary activation
• lateral deltoids
• triceps brachii
• trapezius
• rhomboids
• rectus abdominis
• erector spinae

PROPER FORM
Do
• Perform slow and controlled repetitions
• Keep your torso stabilized and your spine elongated.
• Keep the bar in front of your shoulders.

Avoid
• A partial range of motion.
• Pressing behind your neck
• Arching your back.

MODIFICATIONS
Beginner
• Use a lighter weight.

Advanced
• Use a close underhand grip.

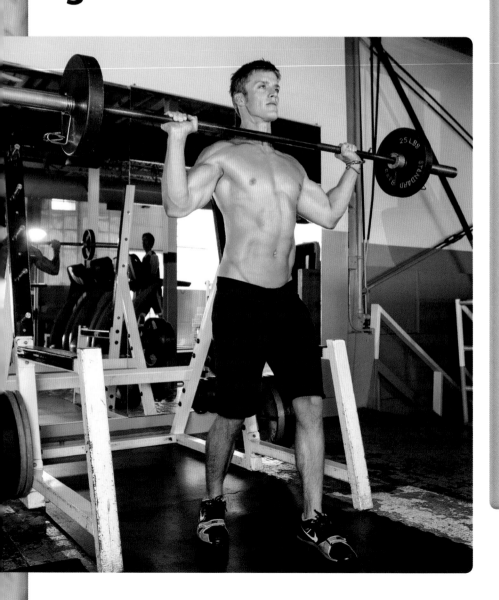

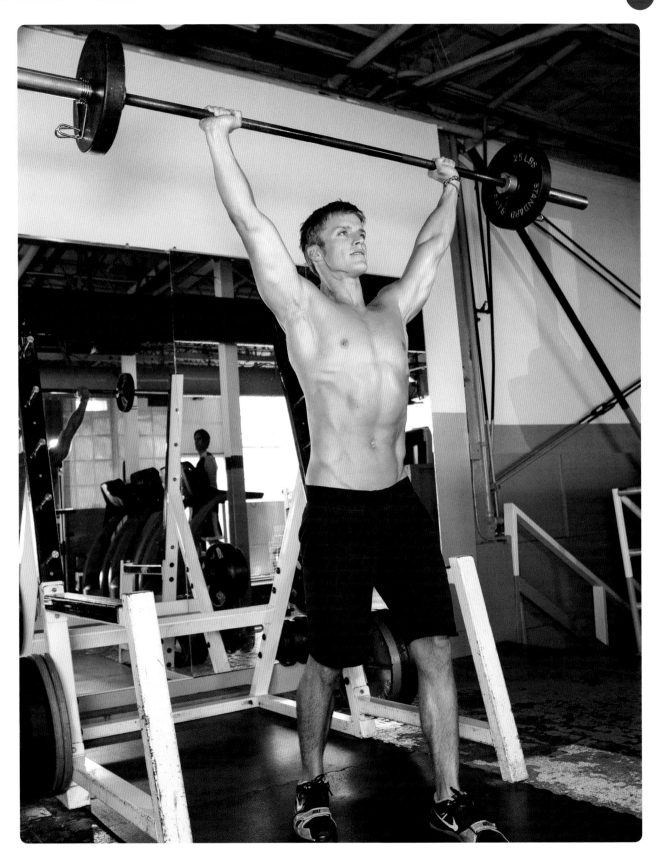

BARBELL POWER CLEAN

PROGRESSION

1 Begin by standing with your arms fully extended while holding a barbell with a wide, overhand grip.

2 Flip the bar as if ducking under it, until it is nearly touching your upper chest.

3 Reverse, and return to the starting position for 6 to 8 repetitions.

MUSCLE ACTION
Primary activation
- deltoids
- triceps brachii
- trapezius

Ancillary activation
- rectus abdominis
- erector spinae
- rhomboids
- gastrocnemius
- soleus

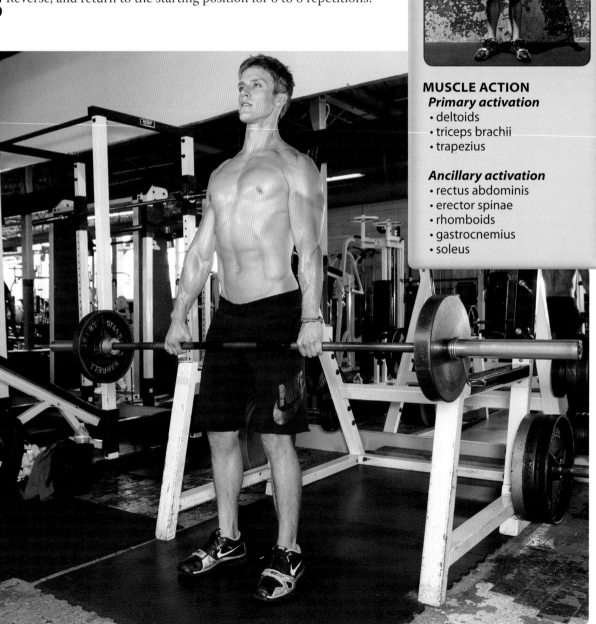

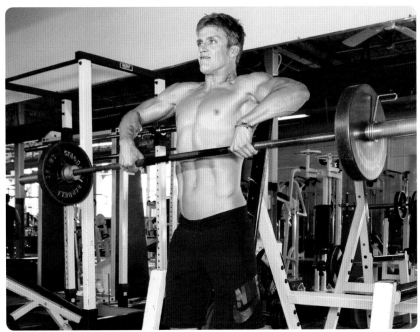

PROPER FORM
Do
- Keep your body stabilized.
- Keep the bar close to your body.
- Move through a full and controlled range of motion.

Avoid
- Overarching your back.
- Too much stress on your wrists.
- Excessive momentum.

MODIFICATIONS
Beginner
- Use a lighter weight.

Advanced
- Use dumbbells.

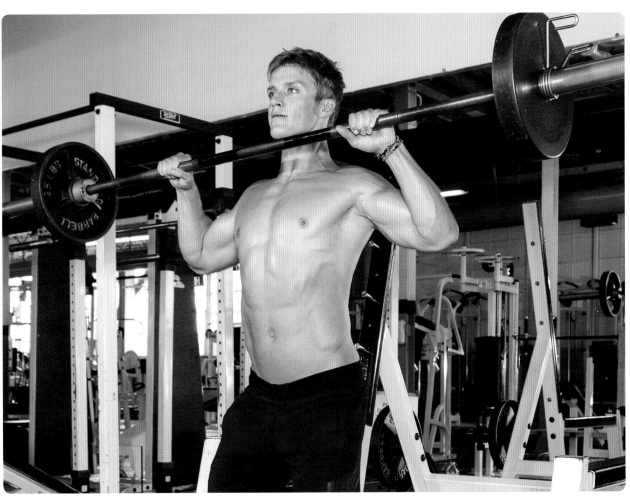

KETTLEBELL ONE-ARM CLEAN AND PRESS

PROGRESSION

1 Begin standing while holding a kettlebell in one hand.

2 Flip the kettlebell up until it is nearly touching your shoulder.

3 Rotate your palm frontward as you simultaneously push overhead. Reverse, and return to the starting position for 6 to 8 repetitions per side.

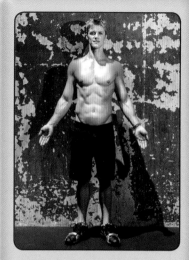

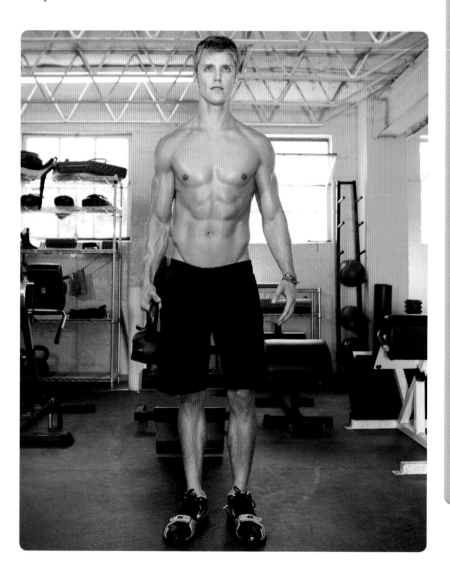

MUSCLE ACTION
Primary activation
- deltoids
- triceps brachii
- trapezius

Ancillary activation
- rectus abdominis
- erector spinae
- rhomboids
- gastrocnemius
- soleus

PROPER FORM
Do
- Keep your body stabilized.
- Keep the kettlebell close to your body.
- Move through a full and controlled range of motion.

Avoid
- Overarching your back.
- Placing too much stress on your wrists.
- Excessive momentum.

MODIFICATIONS
Beginner
- Use a lighter weight.

Advanced
- Lift a kettlebell in each hand.

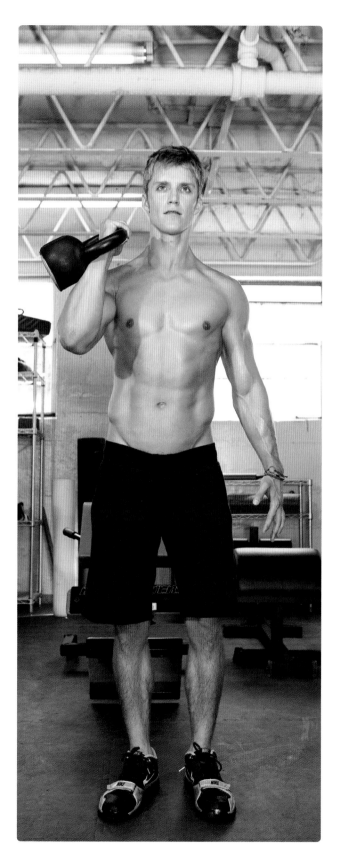
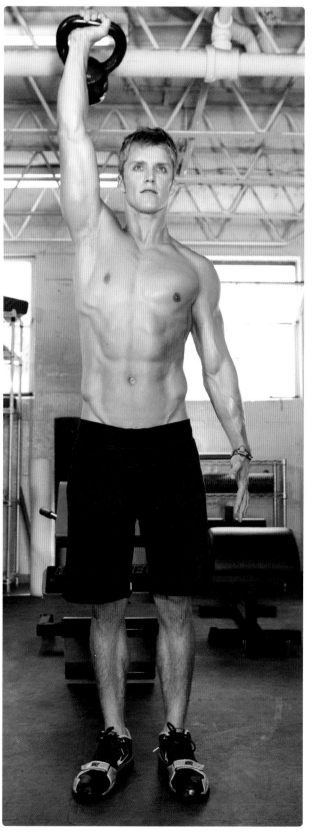

KETTLEBELL ONE-ARM CLEAN

PROGRESSION

1 Begin by bending forward with a flat back and bent knees while holding a kettlebell in one arm. Place the other hand on your thigh for support.

2 Stand tall as you simultaneously flip the kettlebell up until it is nearly touching your shoulder.

3 Reverse, and then return to the starting position. Complete 6 to 8 repetitions, and then repeat on the other side.

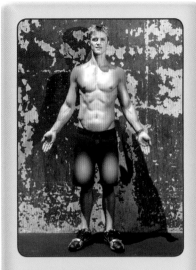

MUSCLE ACTION
Primary activation
- deltoids
- triceps brachii
- trapezius

Ancillary activation
- quadriceps
- gluteus maximus
- rectus abdominis
- erector spinae
- rhomboids
- gastrocnemius
- soleus

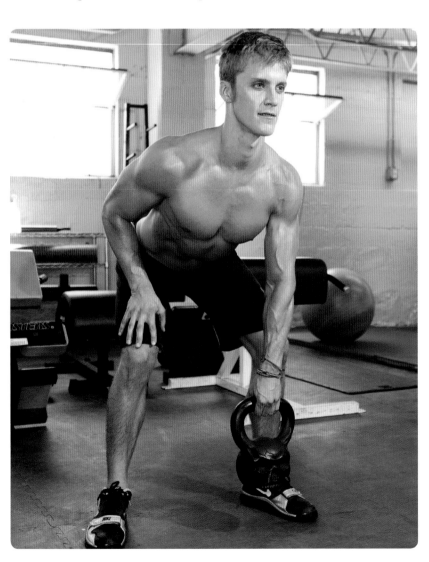

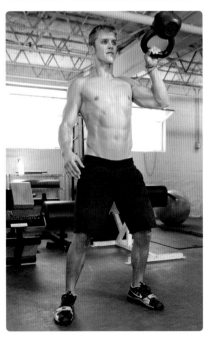

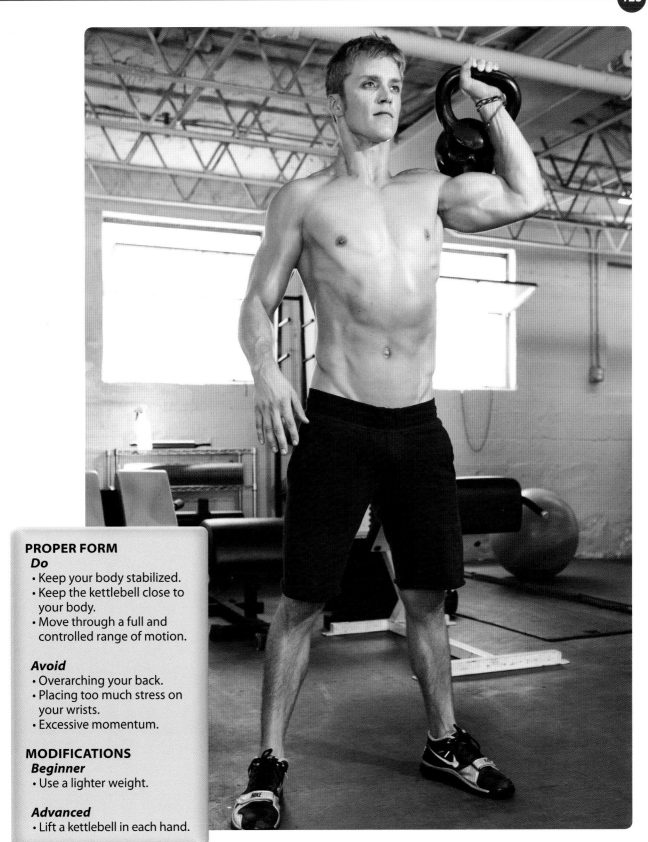

PROPER FORM
Do
- Keep your body stabilized.
- Keep the kettlebell close to your body.
- Move through a full and controlled range of motion.

Avoid
- Overarching your back.
- Placing too much stress on your wrists.
- Excessive momentum.

MODIFICATIONS
Beginner
- Use a lighter weight.

Advanced
- Lift a kettlebell in each hand.

DUMBBELL SHRUG

PROGRESSION

1 Begin in a standing position with your arms extended downward holding a pair of dumbbells at your sides.

2 Lift your shoulders straight up toward your ears.

3 Lower, and repeat for 6 to 10 repetitions.

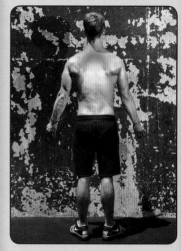

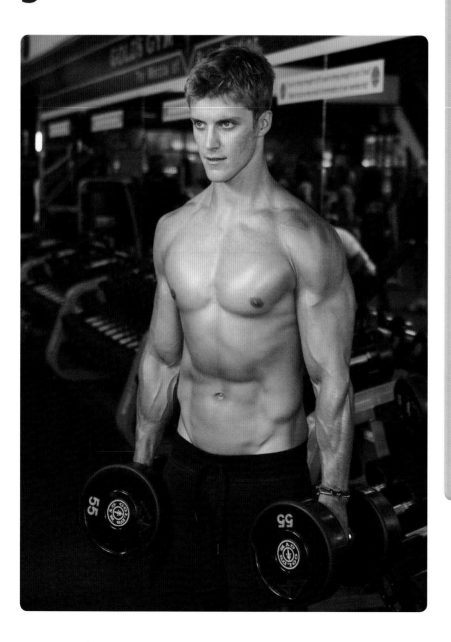

MUSCLE ACTION
Primary activation
- trapezius

Ancillary activation
- rhomboids
- wrist and forearm flexors
- wrist and forearm extensors

PROPER FORM
Do
- Maintain a firm grip.
- Keep the dumbbells close to your sides.
- Elevate your shoulders as high as possible.

Avoid
- Rotating the shoulders.
- Speedy repetitions.
- Allowing the dumbbells to travel around the body.

MODIFICATIONS
Beginner
- Use a lighter weight.

Advanced
- Use a barbell.

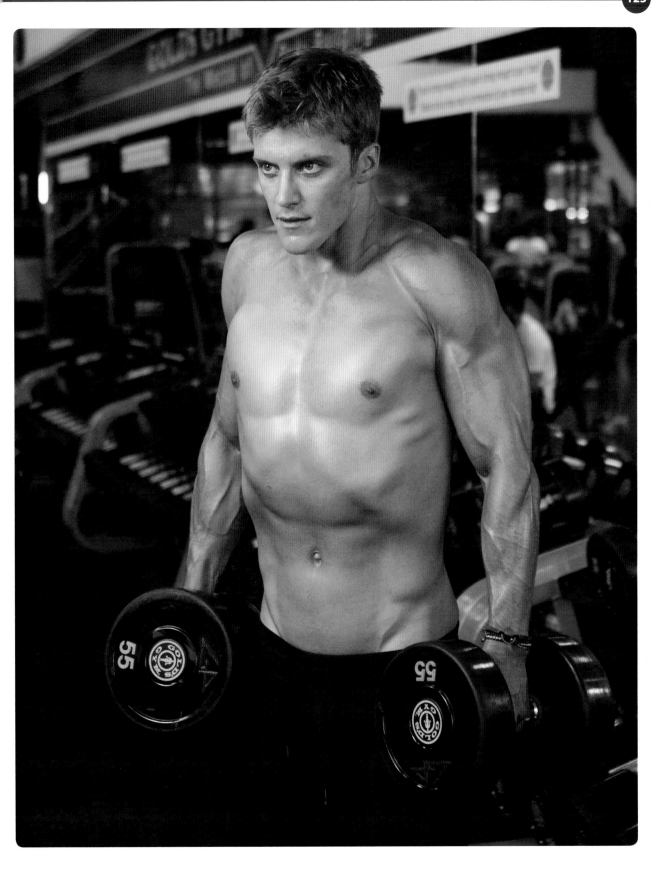

SEATED LATERAL RAISE

PROGRESSION

1 Begin in a seated position with your arms extended down at your sides holding a pair of dumbbells in each hand with your palms facing inward.

2 Bend your arms slightly, and raise them directly out to the side, turning your thumbs downward as you raise your arms parallel to the ground.

3 Lower, and repeat for 8 to 10 repetitions.

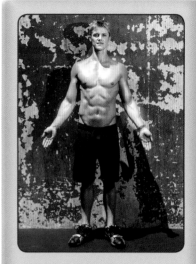

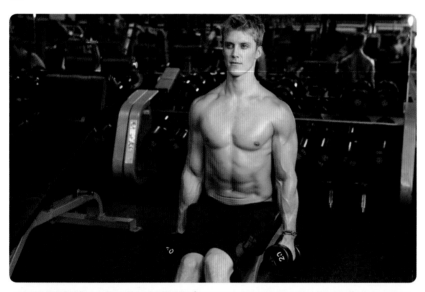

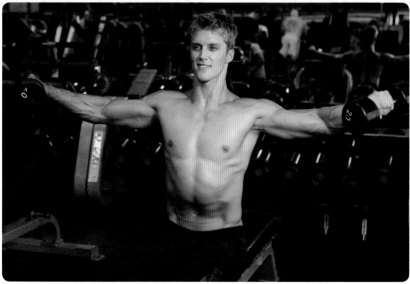

MUSCLE ACTION
Primary activation
• medial deltoids

Ancillary activation
• trapezius
• rhomboids
• wrist and forearm flexors
• wrist and forearm extensors

PROPER FORM
Do
• Maintain a firm grip.
• Maintain proper posture throughout the exercise.
• Point your thumbs slightly downward as you raise your arms.

Avoid
• Raising your arms above parallel to the ground.
• Excessive speed or momentum.
• Keeping your arms straight throughout the exercise.

MODIFICATIONS
Beginner
• Use a lighter weight.

Advanced
• Alternate arms.

BENT-OVER LATERAL RAISE

PROGRESSION

1 Begin standing while holding a pair of dumbbells at your sides. Bend at the knees and lean forward while maintaining a flat back.

2 Raise your arms directly out to the sides in a reverse hugging motion. Return, and repeat for 8 to 10 repetitions.

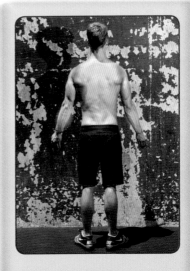

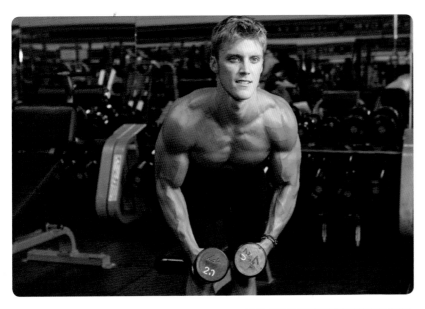

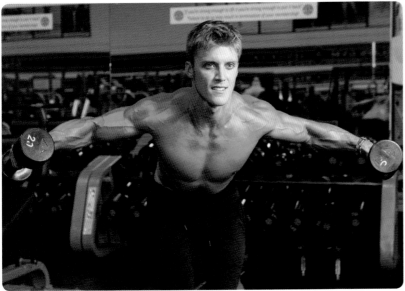

MUSCLE ACTION
Primary activation
- posterior deltoids

Ancillary activation
- trapezius
- rhomboids
- wrist and forearm flexors
- wrist and forearm extensors

PROPER FORM
Do
- Maintain a flat back throughout the movement.
- Keep your arms slightly bent throughout the exercise.
- Move through an arc-like range of motion.

Avoid
- Excessive speed or momentum.
- Rounding your back.
- Allowing your elbows to drop lower than your wrists.

MODIFICATIONS
Beginner
- Use a lighter weight.

Advanced
- Alternate arms.

STANDING SINGLE-ARM LATERAL RAISE

PROGRESSION

1 Begin in a standing position in a cable station with a handle set to the bottom, while holding a pulley in one hand.

2 Bend your arm slightly, and raise it directly out to the side, turning your thumb downward as you raise your arm parallel to the ground. Lower, and repeat for 10 to 12 repetitions per side.

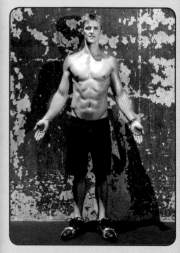

MUSCLE ACTION
Primary activation
• medial deltoids

Ancillary activation
• trapezius
• rhomboids
• wrist and forearm flexors
• wrist and forearm extensors

PROPER FORM
Do
• Maintain proper posture throughout the exercise.
• Keep your arm slightly bent throughout the exercise.
• Point your thumb slightly downward as you raise your arm.

Avoid
• Raising your arm above parallel to the ground.
• Excessive speed or momentum.
• Allowing your elbow to drop lower than your wrist.

MODIFICATIONS
Beginner
• Use a lighter weight.

Advanced
• Use two handles.

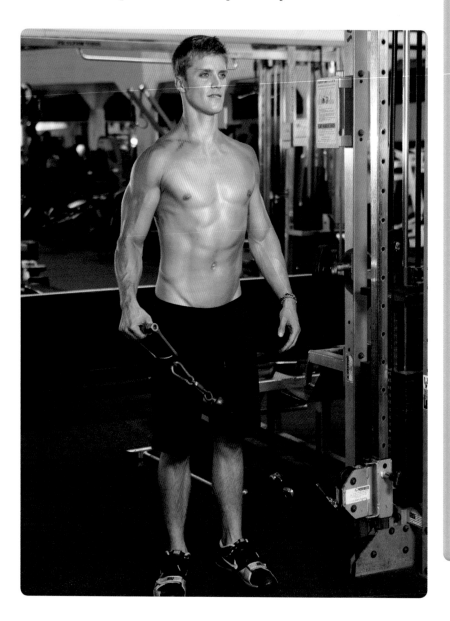

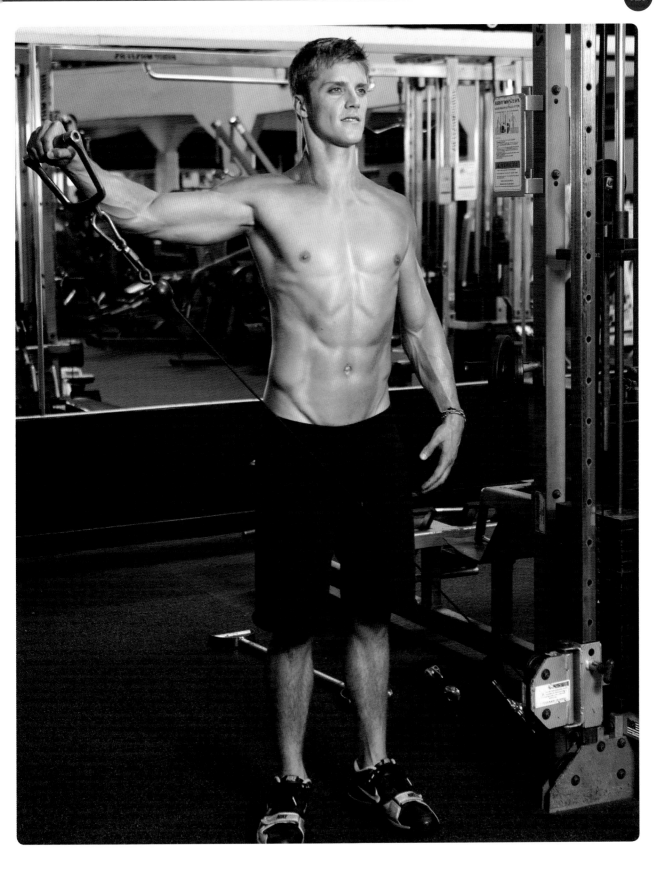

TRICEPS TIPS

Although far less glamorous and noteworthy than the biceps, the triceps brachii muscles are the true key to bigger arms because they compose roughly two-thirds of the upper-arm circumference. When performing triceps exercises, it is important to keep your elbows in and to move through a full range of motion for their complete development.

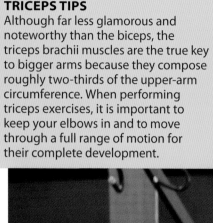

BAR PUSHDOWN

PROGRESSION

1 Begin by standing in front of a cable stack with a bar attached to the top pulley.

2 Take a close grip on the bar, and keep your elbows at your sides with your forearms parallel to the ground.

3 Push straight down until your arms are fully locked, and then raise your arms back to the starting position. Complete 10 to 12 repetitions.

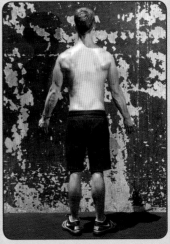

MUSCLE ACTION
Primary activation
- triceps brachii

Ancillary activation
- rhomboids
- rectus abdominis
- erector spinae

PROPER FORM
Do
- Perform slow and controlled repetitions.
- Keep your elbows in at your sides.
- Move through a full and controlled range of motion.

Avoid
- Excessive speed.
- A partial range of motion.
- Flaring your elbows out.

MODIFICATIONS
Beginner
- Use a lighter weight.

Advanced
- Use an underhand or reverse grip.

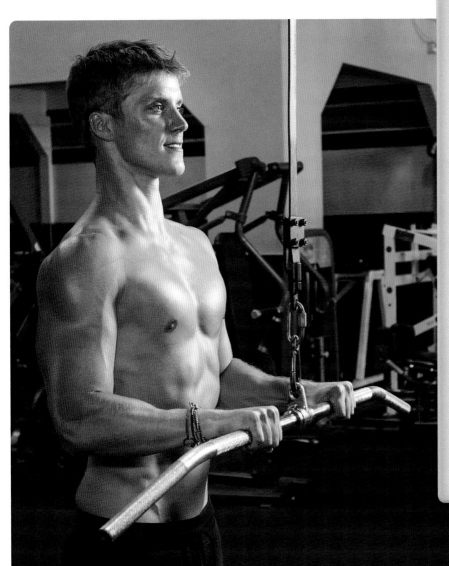

VERTICAL DIP

PROGRESSION

1 Begin by standing in front of a dip station with your hands placed firmly on the ends of the bars. Cross your legs as you lower yourself, leaning back and bending your upper arms until your triceps are parallel to the ground.

2 Push yourself up to lockout, and repeat for 8 to 10 repetitions.

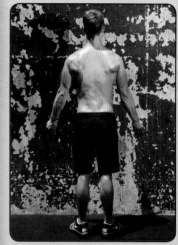

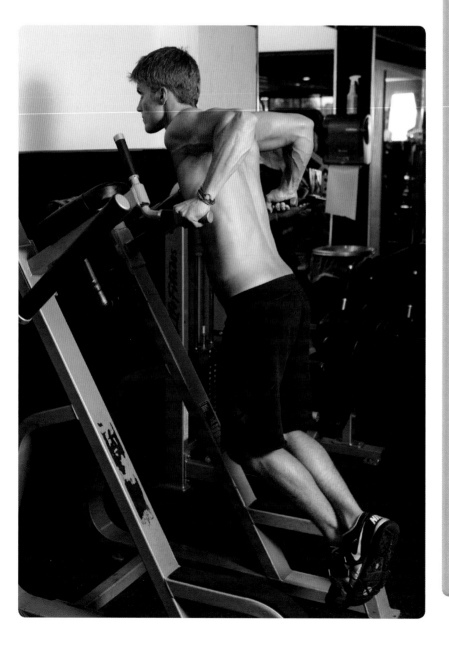

MUSCLE ACTION
Primary activation
• triceps brachii

Ancillary activation
• anterior deltoids
• pectoralis major
• rhomboids
• rectus abdominis

PROPER FORM
Do
• Perform controlled repetitions.
• Keep your upper body straight and your torso stabilized.
• Lower yourself until your upper arms are parallel to the ground.

Avoid
• Excessive speed.
• Shallow or bouncy repetitions.
• Leaning too far forward.

MODIFICATIONS
Beginner
• Have someone assist you at your legs.

Advanced
• Drape chains around your neck for added resistance.

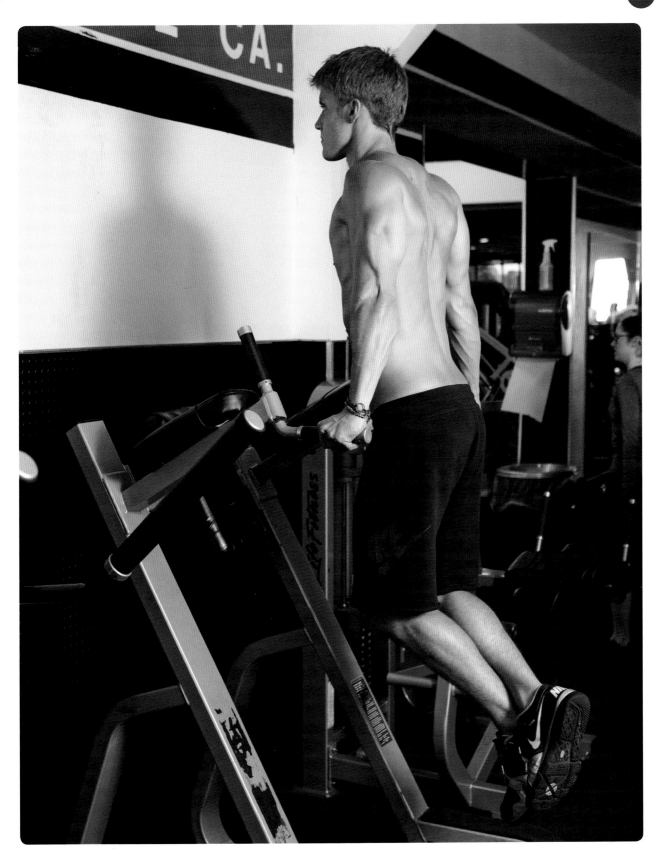

DUMBBELL SKULL CRUSHER

PROGRESSION

1 Begin by lying on your back on a flat bench. Hold a pair of dumbbells at full extension directly over your chest with your palms facing in.

2 Bend your arms backward at the elbow, past your head.

3 Keeping your elbows in and locked in place, extend the dumbbells back up to full lockout over your chest. Repeat for 8 to 10 repetitions.

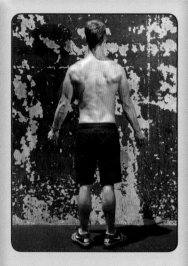

MUSCLE ACTION
Primary activation
- triceps brachii

Ancillary activation
- anterior deltoids
- pectoralis major
- rectus abdominis

PROPER FORM
Do
- Achieve a full stretch behind your head.
- Keep your torso stabilized.
- Keep your elbows in.

Avoid
- Excessive speed.
- Knocking yourself in the head.
- Flaring your elbows.

MODIFICATIONS
Beginner
- Use a barbell.

Advanced
- Use one arm at a time.

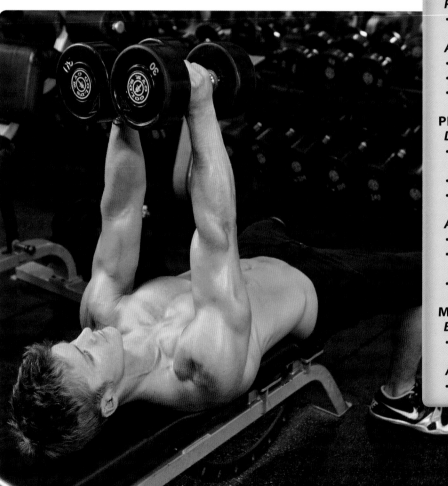

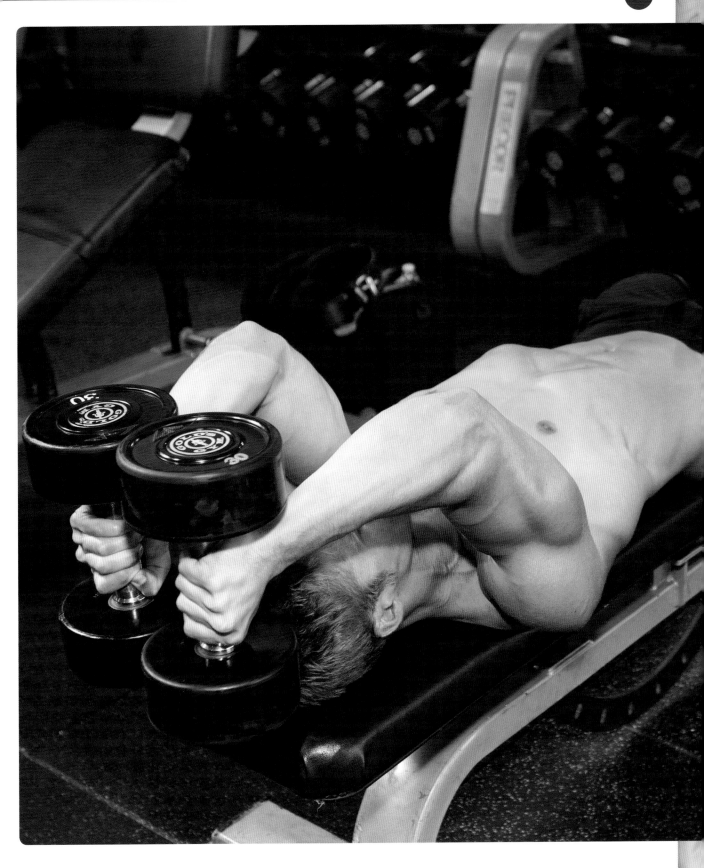

OVERHEAD ROPE EXTENSION

PROGRESSION

1 Begin by standing away from a cable stack with a rope attachment on the top pulley.

2 Grab the rope with both hands, and lean forward maintaining a flat back with a staggered stance. Bend your forearms behind your head while keeping your upper arms locked and your elbows close to your head.

3 Keeping your upper arms stationary, extend your forearms until fully contracted. Repeat for 10 to 12 repetitions.

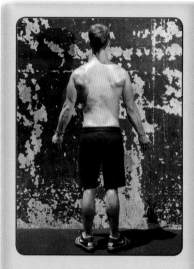

MUSCLE ACTION
Primary activation
- triceps brachii

Ancillary activation
- rhomboids
- rectus abdominis
- erector spinae

PROPER FORM
Do
- Perform slow and controlled repetitions.
- Keep your elbows in and close to your head in the start position.
- Pause when your triceps are fully stretched.

Avoid
- Excessive speed.
- Moving your upper arms.
- Flaring your elbows.

MODIFICATIONS
Beginner
- Use a lighter weight.

Advanced
- Use one arm at a time.

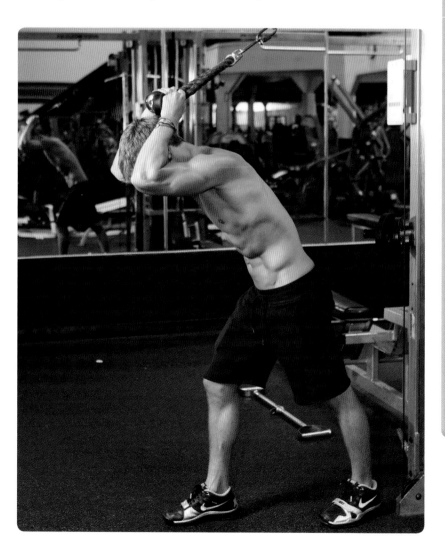

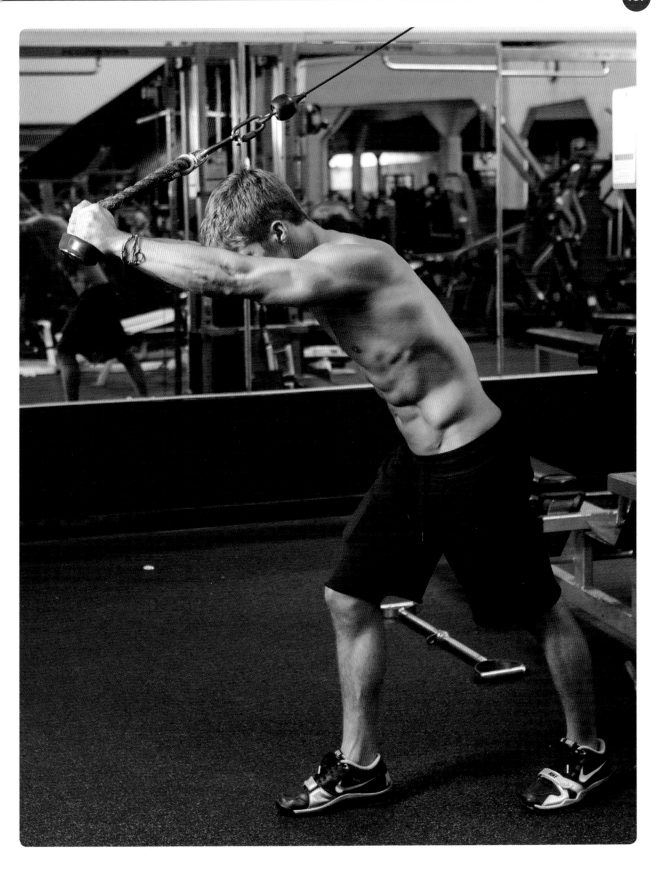

MACHINE TRICEPS EXTENSION

PROGRESSION

1 Begin by sitting in a triceps machine with your upper arms resting on the pad and your hands on the grips, with palms facing in, your arms bent, and your elbows in.

2 Start by extending the arms downward until fully extended. Return to the starting position, and repeat for 10 to 12 repetitions.

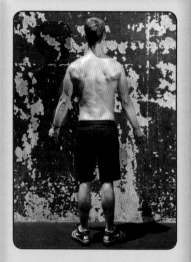

MUSCLE ACTION
Primary activation
- triceps brachii

Ancillary activation
- rectus abdominis
- wrist and forearm flexors
- wrist and forearm extensors

PROPER FORM
Do
- Move through a full range of motion.
- Keep your elbows in.
- Control the weight as you bring it back up.

Avoid
- Allowing your upper arms to lift off the bench.
- Excessive speed or momentum.
- Excessively using your shoulder muscles.

MODIFICATIONS
Beginner
- Use a lighter weight.

Advanced
- Use one arm at a time.

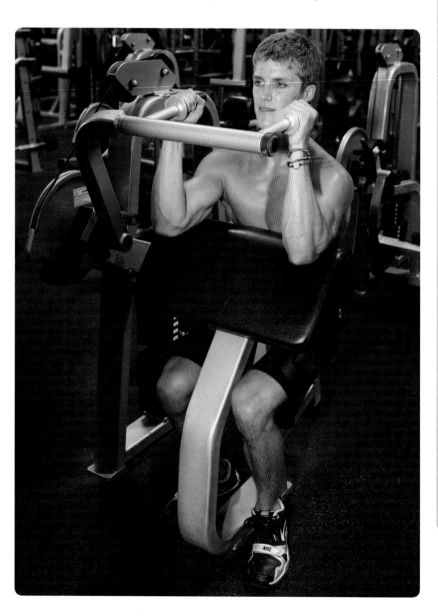

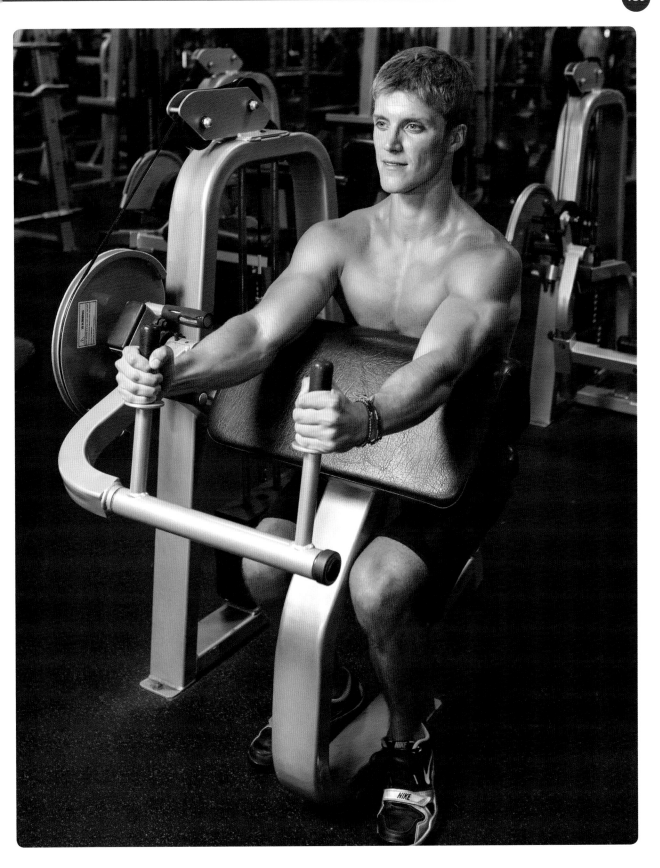

ABDOMINAL TIPS

The abdominal muscles—the rectus abdominis, transversus abdominis, and obliques—support your trunk. It is important to note that the abdominal muscles, particularly the rectus abdominis, are utilized in nearly every exercise imaginable. If you follow this program, they will become strong because of this ancillary use alone. Still, if you are looking for definition, cardio and diet are the keys—even more so than exercise. Having said that, when exercising the abdominals, think of pulling inward from the navel, and not the neck, so as to place and keep the tension on your abs.

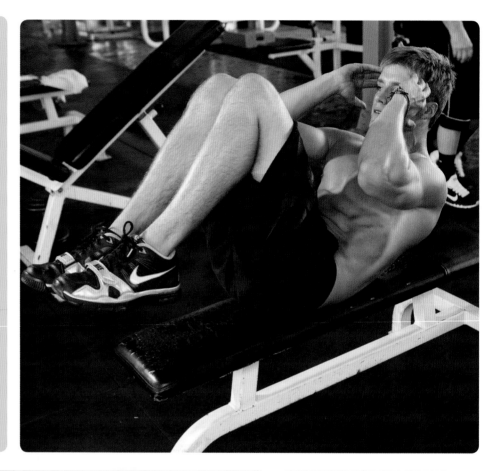

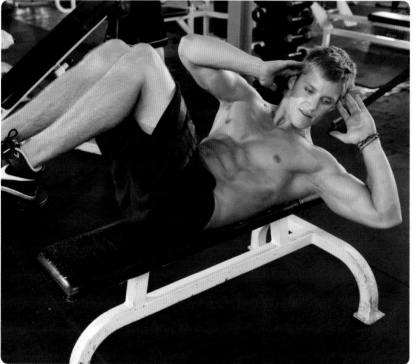

PROPER FORM
Do
- Lead as if pulling from your belly button.
- Contract your abs at the top of the movement.
- Keep your torso stabilized.

Avoid
- Using the neck.
- Speedy or bouncy repetitions.
- Raising your lower back off the bench.

MODIFICATIONS
Beginner
- Keep your feet planted on the bench.

Advanced
- Hold a light dumbbell on your chest.

TWISTING CRUNCH

PROGRESSION

1 Begin by lying back on a flat bench. Bring your knees toward your chest, allowing your feet to dangle in the air. Place your palms on your temples near your ears.

2 Raise your torso toward your knees, and bring one elbow toward the opposite knee.

3 Lower, and alternate sides for 20 repetitions per side.

MUSCLE ACTION
Primary activation
• rectus abdominis
• obliques

Ancillary activation
• erector spinae

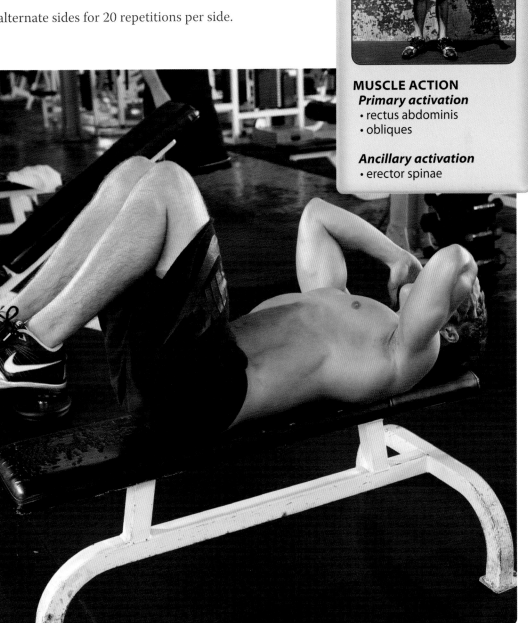

SEATED LEG TUCK

PROGRESSION

1 Sit on a flat bench with your hands gripping the bench by your hips and your legs slightly elevated and bent.

2 Simultaneously bring your legs and torso forward so that your knees meet your chest.

3 Lower in a controlled manner while never allowing your feet to touch the ground, and repeat for 30 repetitions.

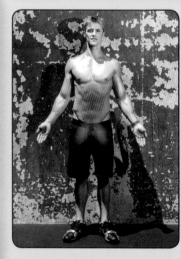

MUSCLE ACTION
Primary activation
- rectus abdominis
- obliques

Ancillary activation
- erector spinae
- hip flexors

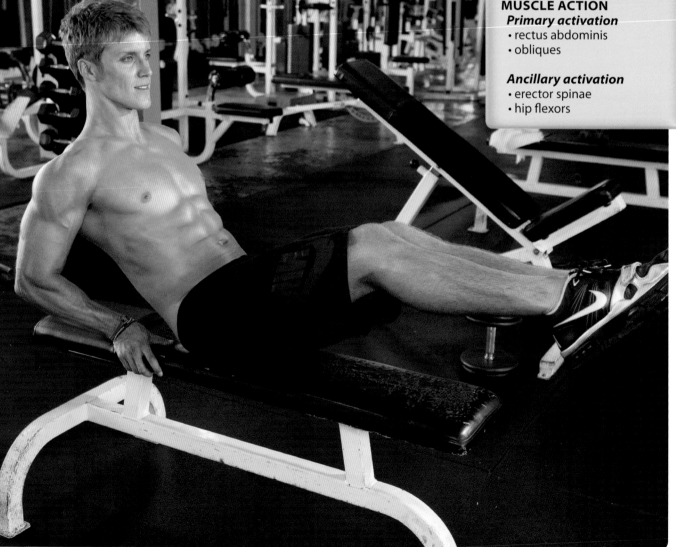

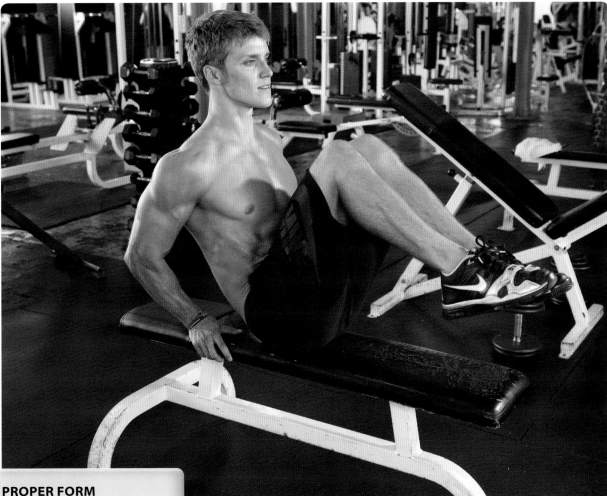

PROPER FORM
Do
- Use a controlled range of motion.
- Use your abdominals to lift.
- Contract your abs at the top of the movement.

Avoid
- Excessive speed.
- A shortened range of motion.
- Arching your back.

MODIFICATIONS
Beginner
- Alternate legs.

Advanced
- Hold a medicine ball between your lower legs.

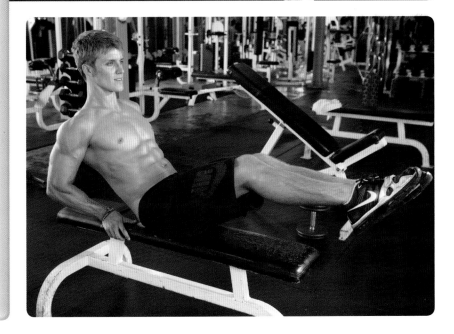

KNEELING LAT STRETCH

PROGRESSION

1 Begin on your knees with your legs bent and your arms outstretched in front and your head tucked in.

2 Lean back to feel the stretch in the latissimus dorsi muscles. Hold for 10 to 30 seconds, and repeat.

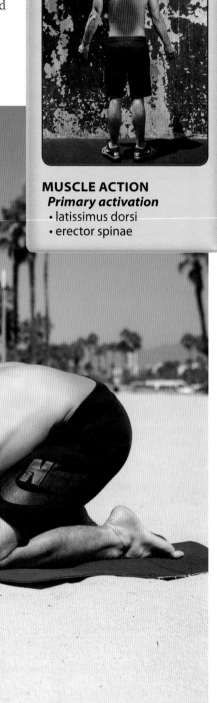

MUSCLE ACTION
Primary activation
- latissimus dorsi
- erector spinae

LOWER-BACK STRETCH

PROGRESSION

1 Begin on your back with your legs bent and your hands clasped around your knees.

2 Gently pull into your chest. Hold for 10 to 30 seconds, and repeat.

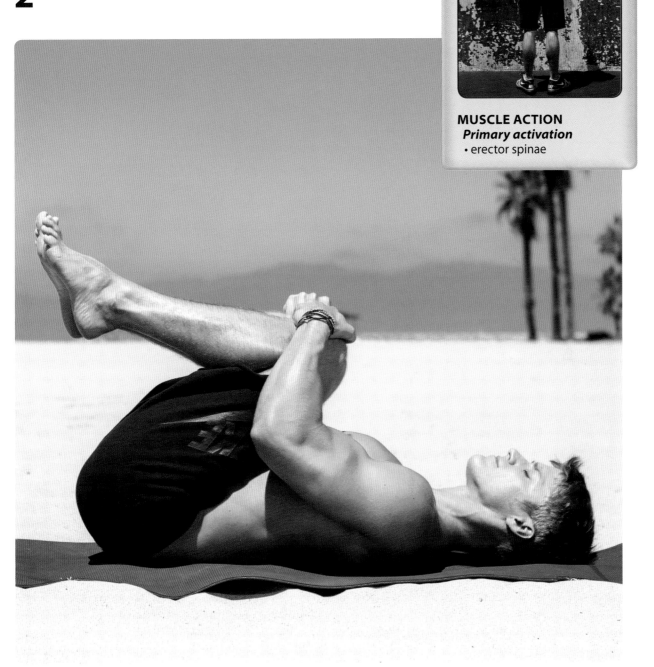

MUSCLE ACTION
Primary activation
• erector spinae

CHEST STRETCH

PROGRESSION

1 Begin in a standing position while facing a corner, and plant your hands on each side of the wall.

2 Gently push your chest forward to feel the stretch in your pectoral muscles. Hold for 10 to 30 seconds, and repeat.

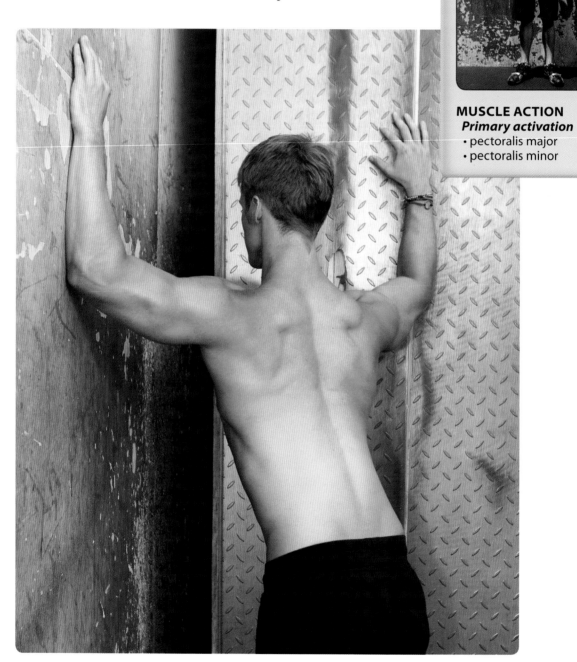

MUSCLE ACTION
Primary activation
- pectoralis major
- pectoralis minor

BICEPS STRETCH

PROGRESSION

1 Begin standing with one arm extended in front of you and your palm facing upward.

2 Using your free hand, gently stretch your fingers backward. Hold for 10 to 30 seconds, and then repeat with the other arm.

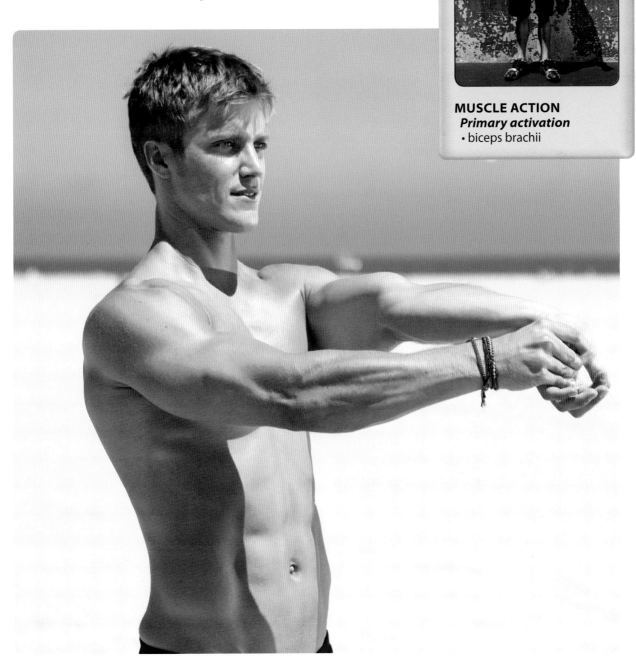

MUSCLE ACTION
Primary activation
• biceps brachii

TOE TOUCH

PROGRESSION

1 Begin in a standing position with your legs as straight as possible.

2 Slowly and with control, bend at the waist, allowing your fingertips to touch the ground.

3 Stretch, and hold for 10 to 30 seconds, and then repeat.

MUSCLE ACTION
Primary activation
- biceps femoris
- semitendinosus
- semimembranosus

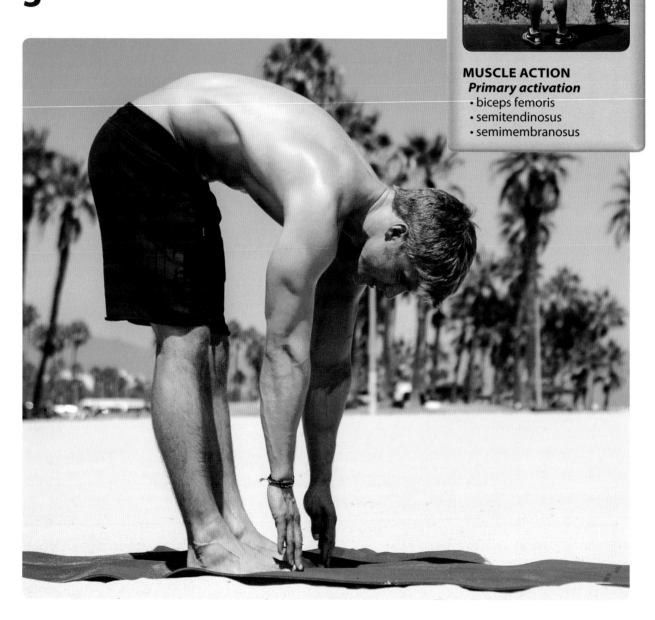

QUAD STRETCH

PROGRESSION

1 Begin seated such that your legs are bent and you are resting your glutes on your feet with your arms behind you for support.

2 Lean back to feel the stretch in your quadriceps.

3 Hold for 10 to 30 seconds, and repeat.

MUSCLE ACTION
Primary activation
- rectus femoris
- vastus lateralis
- vastus intermedius
- vastus medialis

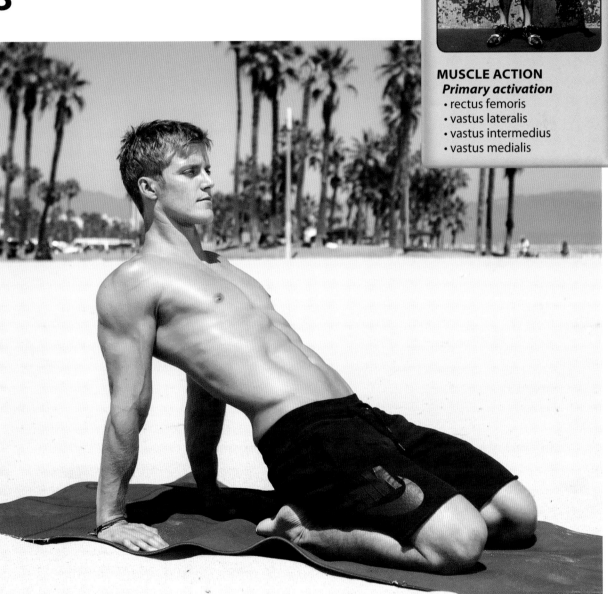

CALF STRETCH

PROGRESSION

1 Begin in a standing position with one foot flat on the ground and the other raised on a step or platform.

2 Stretch your heel down toward the ground, and raise your toes.

3 Hold for 10 to 30 seconds, and repeat with the other foot.

MUSCLE ACTION
Primary activation
- gastrocnemius
- soleus

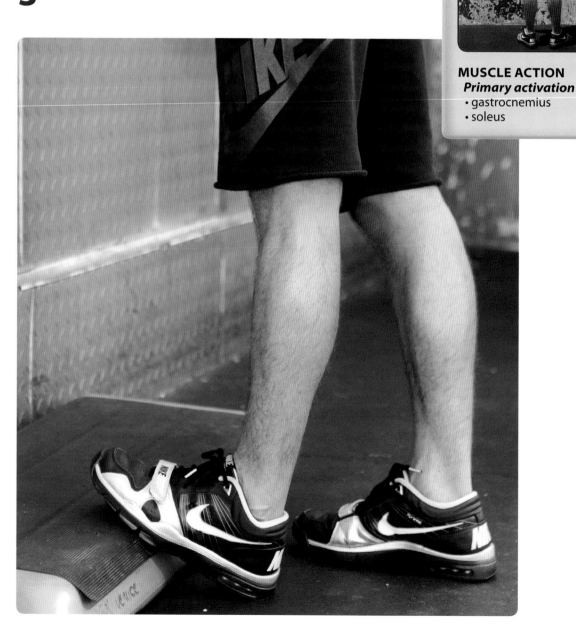

SHOULDER STRETCH

PROGRESSION

1 Begin in a seated position with your legs bent, your chest out, and your arms behind you for support with your fingers pointing away from you.

2 Stick out your chest while maintaining an erect posture.

3 Hold for 10 to 30 seconds, and repeat.

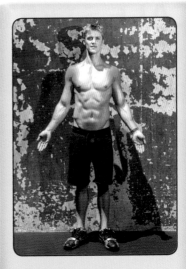

MUSCLE ACTION
Primary activation
• deltoids

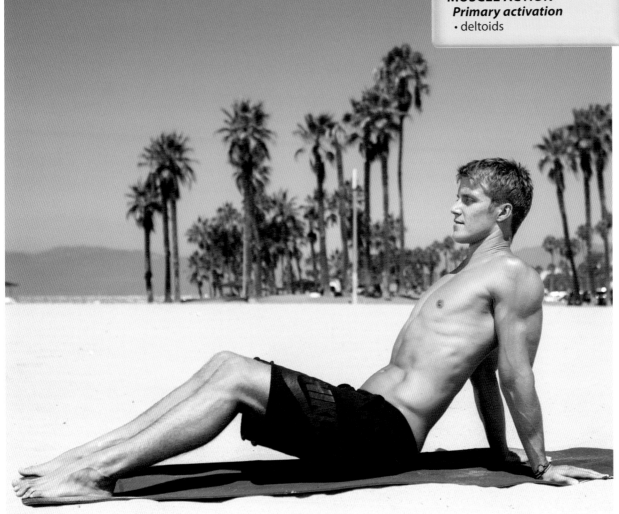

TRICEPS STRETCH

PROGRESSION

1 Begin in a standing position with one arm behind your back holding one end of a towel and your other arm parallel to your head holding the other end of the towel.

2 Bend your overhead arm to a 90-degree angle while holding the towel tightly between your arms with little, if any, slack. Feel the stretch in the triceps.

3 Hold for 10 to 30 seconds, and repeat with the opposite arm.

MUSCLE ACTION
Primary activation
• triceps brachii

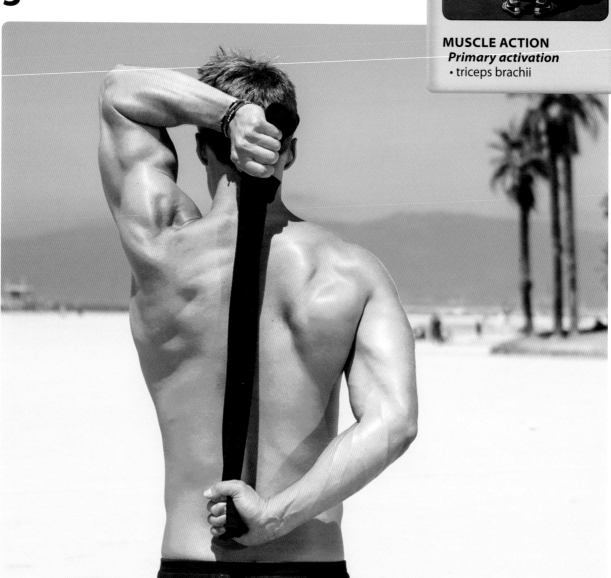

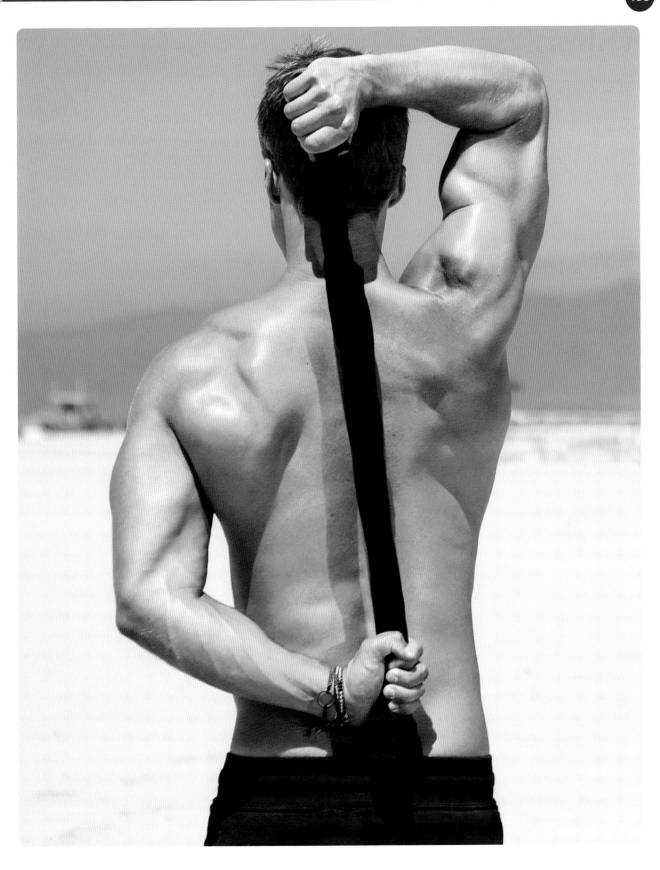

THE HUMAN CONDITION

For many of us, the possibilities of the journey, the allure, is what draws our attention. It's that magic moment before signing on the dotted line. It's that indescribable feeling that happens when the dice soar through the air. How many times have you sought out something only to quickly attain it and then put it down? That new car smell and careful shutting of the door soon leads to coffee stains and items thrown about.

Recently I bought a guitar because music is a huge part of my life, and I always wanted to learn to play some of the songs I listen to when I workout. I played the guitar every day at first, but soon I went days without even picking it up. When so many friends kept asking me how my guitar playing was going, I sought the only way I could to feed the initial passion and get myself back on track: lessons. Because the truth is, this goal is important to me. I *can* make the time to learn this instrument. It's never fun when others ask, "How's that goal going?" and we have to answer, "It's not," knowing that we've given up.

Indeed for many of us, life often gets in the way, creating a barrier between us and our goals. And then we realize just how difficult the task ahead truly is. In their quest for size, countless ectomorphs give up somewhere along the road because gains seem too hard to come by, or the amount of effort applied does not seem to warrant the results garnered. Even if the human tendency or condition is more often than not to give up, you still have the power to take a stand, make a decision and, ultimately, make a change. It starts with blocking out that lazy, passive voice in your head that whispers, "You can't do this," and then listening to the other voice that screams, "Yes you can. Now go!"

I have been on dates where my alarm went off, and in the middle of some sort of mutual activity, I've pulled out a Tupperware meal from under the car seat much to the surprise of the girl next to me because I had to get meal five in. I have sat through college lectures barely listening and mentally plotting that day's leg workout, and then excusing myself from class for five minutes so I could scarf down a meal. I would then have to explain to the class when put on the spot about my reasons for stepping out. My answer was, "Because I'm the one on stage in a few months in my underwear posing in front of hundreds of people, and I want to be improved from my last appearance on stage, and I want to win!"

Maybe I took things to the extreme, but you can clearly see my dedication—I wanted to win that badly, and nothing would stop me from my goals. I was constantly motivated—obsessed even—with bettering my physique from my last show. And my life has always been set up in priorities to get my goals accomplished. Getting in my training, meals, and ample recuperation remain firmly in the pole position and, as a result, I have complete mastery over my body. And so too will you!

Negative people may try to put you and your efforts down. Pay them no mind because this journey is a personal one. Be thankful that you do not have to rely on them. Never let the other guy's belief that *he* can't reach a goal make you believe that *you* can't. We all have insecurities, but if you prep meticulously, those insecurities are eclipsed by success.

We run much harder when someone is chasing us. And even more powerfully when that "someone" is really "you," chasing after a new best. Set your own standard, and refuse to accept anything less than results. Remember, validation lives in self-approval. You started this journey and continue on for you.

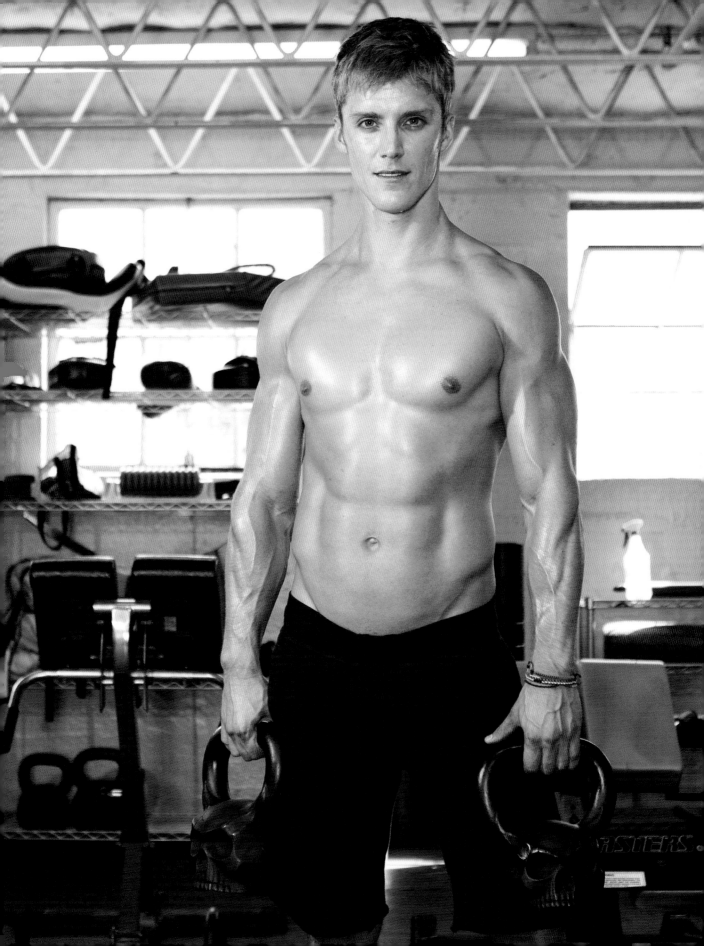

CONDITIONS TO SUCCESS

If you think of each step to ensure your progress as a bolt in a track, then the track is sturdy and ensures a smooth and steady trek by the train. We are talking specifically about physical actions that will help to keep your mental "eye of the tiger" and keep you on track (pun intended) and progressing.

Packing. Packing meals in advance is instrumental in getting you closer to your physique goals. I rarely, if ever, leave my house for the day without a few meals in my car. This helps to ensure I don't miss meals and blow my program, especially if I'm in a place that has very limited options.

Danger Zone. Go where you can't help but measure your progress, like the beach or the pool—places where your shirt comes off, and you are forced to show how your far along you are on your muscle-building journey.

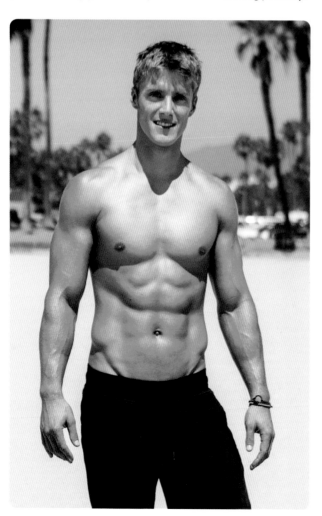

Future Glory. Post a picture of you at your current best somewhere you will see it frequently, perhaps on your fridge door. Look at it with the thought that you are going to best that physique going forward. Improvement is the ever-present goal.

Recruits. Although bodybuilding is largely an individual effort, sometimes keeping yourself on track is easier when you share the journey. My good friend lives across the country but was getting ready for his second bodybuilding contest while I was outlining this book and getting myself into shape for another. We constantly kept each other up to date on our progress in an honest and constructive manner. He even helped me one night in particular when I really wanted a cheat meal but was too close to the photo shoot to allow myself that indulgence. He talked me down, so to speak. Friends have each others' backs and can truly make a difference.

Those Who Have Been There. Watching some of my favorite bodybuilders' videos on YouTube and training videos has always helped to keep me motivated and on the highway toward future progress. I guarantee that there is someone out there you'd love to look like. Use his videos for motivation, inspiration, perspiration, and, ultimately, muscle regeneration.

TAKE, DON'T ASK

It is your dream, and no doubt you want it. If you have this book in your hands, you're probably thinking, "Finally, someone is speaking to me!" This was the recurring thought in my head as I planned and wrote this book. Time and time again I have personally inspected the training section in local bookstores and even searched online and rarely, if ever, found a resource that speaks directly to the seemingly ignored and invisible ectomorphic audience. So the chances are likely that your motivation is running high, your allegiance to yourself has been renewed, and you are more than ready for this journey—done the right way. But should your motivation wane (which is the normal human condition), please allow me to share a personal story.

There was a local park near my parents' house. It wasn't particularly big or elaborate; it was merely a baseball field with weeds and undeveloped acres directly behind it that seemed to go on forever. Beyond outfield was a fence that led into a neighborhood. One day I brought a bat and a couple of balls. I tossed the ball in the air and swung. Missed. Tossed again. A small hit. Fast forward many weeks . . . many, many weeks.

I became almost obsessed with hitting the ball over the fence just one single time. I'd come close with many high-poppers that seemed to go up into outer space merely to descend and drop back down mere feet from the fence. I tried and tried hundreds upon hundreds of times. No matter what, I would not quit. I would somehow, some way, one day hit the ball over. This went on for months in my own private war. My sides hurt from the jarring twisting. My hands were cut up from the gripping. And my head was hurting from the mental torment I put myself through. Soon, I was planning to move out on my own and venture into the world. I didn't care. I would return home and hit that ball over.

There comes a point in every journey where the protagonist nears the finish line and questions the "why" of his quest as the odds against him surmount. I was at that point. So close with so many attempts and misses, yet that journey was unfinished. And for whatever the reason, I remembered why that goal was so important to me. And then one day, on an otherwise not particularly magnificent day, I tossed the ball up, took a mighty swing, and made the "crack" sound as bat makes perfect connection with the ball. Maybe it was the force, speed, angle, wind, or just pity from above, but that ball went sailing, easily passing over the fence. I could have cried. In fact, my eyes welled up. Dreams: never give up!

At that particular time, the baseball diamond was my war. Right now, the gym is your personal battlefield where waging war yields a better you.

MEASURING PROGRESS . . . AND BEYOND

The report card. The work evaluation. The bank statement. These are all means of measuring progress. Where we are in the grand scheme of things is always in flight, always in flux, always changing. In terms of bodybuilding, this need to measure progress is no different. It might even seem uber-important to check your progress because of the sometimes demanding lifestyle that is associated with freeing your genetic limits.

Yet, measuring progress can often stop it in its tracks. One of the top ways to thwart yourself is developing a multiple-times-a-day adherence to checking the scale. Keep off it! Although it searches for homeostasis (constant state of being), the human body is always in flux, and your weight is a constantly changing number. For instance, you're generally going to weigh less in the morning than at night because you've fasted while asleep. Weigh yourself late in the day, after a big meal, and the number will rise.

Contrary to popular belief, however, the hardgainer's journey is far more than numbers. Yes, numbers on macronutrients consumed and numbers on poundages hoisted are important. But it's the intangibles such as recuperation and overall health that can't be measured in numbers that tells the true tale of advancement. If you must weigh yourself, then let it be once per week at the same time of the day. But even this number falls short of the full story—namely your body's composition. If we are talking numbers, the ones that truly matter are how much lean muscle mass you are carrying and your body-fat percentage. Remember, the scale is not your friend, meaning that it will always be honest, and yet not reveal the full story.

This may leave you wondering, how then can I chart my progress? Well, it's your reflection, your clothes, and your increasing target sets that tell a much truer story of your journey.

Unsolicited compliments from fellow gym-goers or impressed friends or relatives whom you haven't seen for a while who ask, "Hey, are you working out?" will sure help reinforce the idea that you have made progress. Yet, tracking progress can start as simply as standing in front of a mirror. Updated photographs, tighter clothes, and increasing poundages as recorded in your training diary are all good indicators of positive change.

THE NEW YOU

Congratulations! You've made it this far in your journey. In any endeavor, no matter how much you progress, it is human nature to always want to better yourself. And no matter how much you progress, there will be someone who has progressed further. It really doesn't matter, though, because this journey is all about you. Someone may have bigger arms, but you may have thinner skin and more prominent vascularity, giving you the appearance of the better set of arms. Someone else may have wider shoulders, but you may have more detail in your shoulders, making the other guy appear smooth by comparison. It doesn't matter, because we have no control over others, only ourselves. Reaching your own personal ceiling of development is the ultimate payoff. Learning to

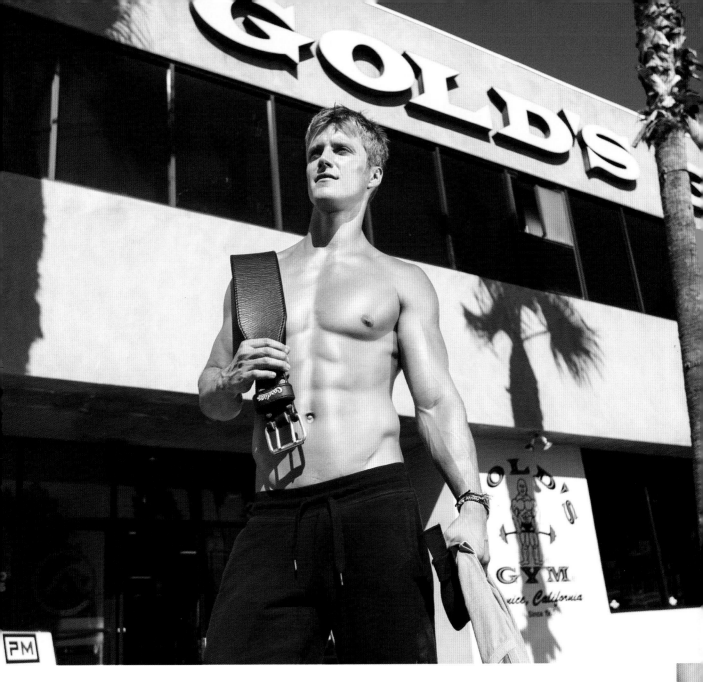

utilize your own genetic strengths and playing to them will serve you throughout your bodybuilding career and even carry over into other aspects of your life.

We are often striving to complete one journey and then set out for another. Too many of us focus on too many possible destinations and never even get going. Once you've reached the 12-week point of this program, you've not reached the end of your journey—it continues on, indefinitely. There is no limit to human development. Your ultimate self hasn't yet been revealed because it is constantly in motion, improving. As long as desire remains as constant as a beating heart, then you can always get one more rep or lift more weight than you have previously, and you can continue to improve. Having

said that, reaching the 12-week mark with this program is a huge achievement. Compare the pictures taken when you first undertook this journey (You did remember to take them, didn't you? I thought so . . .) with the image that stares back at you in the mirror right now, and I dare you to tell me you can't see improvement.

With that, go to the beach, take your shirt off, and be proud. Go to a park in that tank top and show off those arms. Or even go on a date wearing a form-fitting shirt (athletic cut, of course) that showcases your new V taper. Just maybe—just maybe—on your way you'll see someone very familiar. Someone who closely resembles the you of just a short 12 weeks ago. And let him know that there is indeed hope and a way.

ABOUT THE AUTHOR

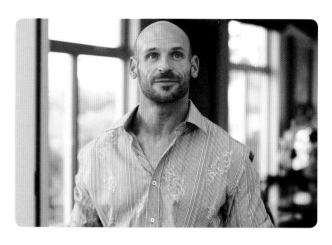

Before his career as author and personal trainer, HOLLIS LANCE LIEBMAN had been a fitness magazine editor, national bodybuilding champion, and published physique photographer, and he has also served as a bodybuilding and fitness competition judge. Currently a Los Angeles resident, Hollis has worked with some of Hollywood's elite, earning himself rave reviews. *From Slight to Might* is his tenth book.

Visit www.holliswashere.com to keep up with all of his things social, including fitness tips and complete training programs.

ABOUT THE MODEL

BRIAN BENTLEY is a certified personal trainer and lifestyle coach based out of Los Angeles, California. He has been involved in fitness nearly all his life, beginning with team sports, and then continuing on to a focused, tactical approach to health and body training. After graduating with degrees from the California State University, Northridge, in Recreation Therapy and Sport and Recreation Management, he focused his efforts on improving the lives of the residents of his SoCal community. Brian's philosophy on fitness is simple: fitness is fun. Yes, it is difficult—a test of both the body and the mind. But, with the right strategy and mind-set, all of us can overcome challenges and achieve our fitness goals. What isn't fun about that?

Visit his website, brianbentleyfitness.com, for fitness tips, ideas, and plain old fun.

Email: Brian@brianbentleyfitness.com

Instagram: @brianbentleyfit

CREDITS

Editorial and design by Lisa Purcell Editorial & Design (purcelleditorial.com)

Photography by Jen Schmidt (jenschmidtphotography.com)

Female model: Michelle Brooke (www.michellebrooke.com)

Weight belt provided by Cardillo (http://www.cardillousa.com)

Photographed on location at Gold's Gym, Venice, California, USA (www.goldsgym.com/veniceca/), and Fitness Factory L.A., West Hollywood, California, USA (www.fitnessfactoryla.com).

Recipes and food images supplied by The Life Chef (www.lalifechef.com).

All photos by Jen Schmidt, except the following: 12 mflippo/CanStockPhoto; 27 *top left* viperagp/CanStockPhoto; 27 *middle left* Mullookkaaran/Wikimedia Commons; 28 *left* draghicich/CanStockPhoto; 36 Championstudio/CanStockPhoto; 38 uatp1/CanStockPhoto; 40 *left* rimglow/CanStockPhoto; 40 *right* lunamarina/CanStockPhoto

ACKNOWLEDGMENTS

The author wishes to thank the good people of Gold's Gym, Venice, California; Fitness Factory L.A., West Hollywood, California; and especially the tireless efforts of Lisa Purcell and Jen Schmidt.

This book is dedicated to the true hardgainer, the ectomorph. May this book duly illuminate your journey, take you further than you've ever been, and finally deliver to you the ultimate satisfaction in the gym, on the beach, and most important, in the mirror.